What people are saying about *Shape Shifting . . .*

Just as you promised, I have found your writing to be "easy to read," and free of confusing jargon and medical terminology!

I wasn't expecting it to also be so captivating that I found myself getting lost in enjoying the book and forgetting my purpose of looking for helpful suggestions for you!

Thank you for writing this book and inviting me to be among the first to enjoy it.

Marie Vest
Dream Team Editor

- - - -

Thank you, Sharon, for including me as one of your Dream Team staff!

I've learned so much about you, health, taking care of my own sweet self on many levels in ways I hadn't considered, etc., by reading your book.

This is an awesome book ~ a job masterfully done!

Sherai Boyd
Dream Team Editor

- - - -

Wow, what a difference!

Sharon, I saw you a few weeks back when I was taking an afternoon walk at Unity Village. At first I didn't recognize the tall slender woman strolling by the rose garden fountains, but then I realized it was you! You look awesome and you carry yourself with such grace and ease. Congratulations on your personal shape shifting experience! I know you will touch many lives through sharing your message in speaking engagements and through your book.

Walk on woman!

Rev. Diana Kennedy
www.RevDianaKennedy.com

A supervisor and I were in the breakroom talking about weight loss. Sharon was sitting at a table eating her lunch. I pointed to her and said, "But the Queen of Weight Loss is sitting right there." It seemed for awhile that every time I saw her Sharon had lost more weight. Her "shape shifting" ability has not gone unnoticed in the workplace.

Rev. Crystal Muldrow

Unity of Albany, New York

- - - - -

A very personal book that covers the whole gamut of living healthily.

Barbara Willeford

Dream Team Editor

- - - - -

It was a pleasure reading *Shape Shifting*. Your passion is contagious. Your writing style quickly captivates the reader and takes them on your personal journey. I know this book will be a source of hope and inspiration to many.

Darryl Corcoran

Dream Team Editor

- - - - -

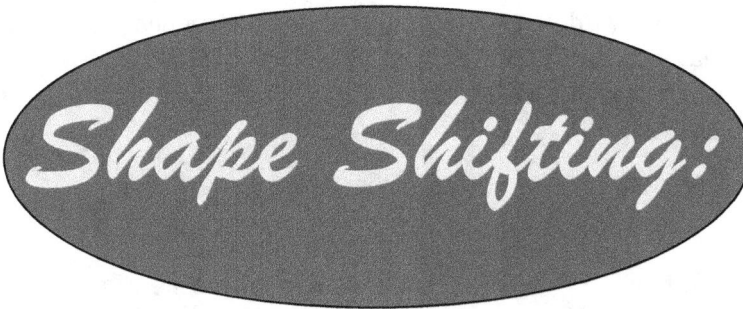

The Alchemy of Losing Weight and Keeping It Off

By Sharon Kay,
M.A., L.U.T.

Write to: Life of Victory Enterprises
                 P. O. Box 1266
                 Lees Summit, MO 64063
E-Mail: Sharon@SharonKays.website

FIRST U.S. EDITION

COVER DESIGN & PHOTOGRAPHY by:
    Dawn Boomsa Photography, Inc.

MOTIVATIONAL COACH & PUBLICIST: Joy Cherry

DREAM TEAM EDITORS:

Barbara Willeford	**Bernadette Swanson**
Carolyn Carter	**Darryl Corcoran**
Joy Cherry	**Marie Vest**
Sherai Boyd	

ISBN-13: 978-1512113686

ISBN-10: 1512113689

LCCN: 2015908103

ACKNOWLEDGEMENTS

It would take several pages to list all Unity ministers, teachers, classmates, coworkers, supervisors, and leaders without whom this book would not exist. Rather than risk offending anyone from past relationships, I have chosen to cite churches, groups, and organizations which had a significant impact on the development of this book.

~ ~ ~ ~ ~ ~ ~

Family and Friends

Unity of Independence, Missouri

Unity of New Braunfels, Texas

Unity of Houston, Texas

Silent Unity Telephone Prayer Ministry

Spiritual Education & Enrichment Program

Licensed Unity Teacher Program

Empowerment Prayer Group

Sceniuses Group

Inner Core Group

Power Posse Group

Weight Watchers

Overeaters Anonymous

~ ~ ~ ~ ~ ~ ~

VISION AND MISSION STATEMENTS

My vision for this book is for every man, woman and child who has ever been told that they are fat to have an opportunity to lean from my experiences. I believe it will make a difference in their lives and in the world's consciousness. Don't tell me it is impossible. I know that one person can change the world.

~ ~ ~ ~ ~ ~ ~

My mission, and your mission, should you decide to accept it, is to see to it that this book gets into the hands of everyone who needs it. There is so much pain in the world and if this one issue, obesity, was addressed appropriately, much of the suffering would be alleviated. If you are one of the people to whom this book is addressed, know that I love you. I empathize with you. But I do not sympathize with or feel sorry for you. The purpose of this book is to empower you, for you have the power within you to change anything about you that is causing you to be less than the beautiful human being you were born to be.

As you will read, I have walked in your shoes. Not only have I been morbidly obese, but I: 1) have been in two abusive marriages; 2) have a bladder with diminished capacity and a diagnosis of Interstitial Cystitis; 3) have lived at poverty-level on Section 8 housing and food stamps; and 4) moved 750 miles with no guarantee of a job, no savings and an income of less than $1,000 a month, leaving family and friends, in order to rise above the welfare state.

So, if you are reading this book, know that you, too, are capable of making tremendous changes to your life. I believe in YOU!

~ ~ ~ ~ ~ ~ ~

"Today I stop placing limits on my ability to live the life of my dreams."

DailyWord magazine, June 14, 2015

Table of Contents

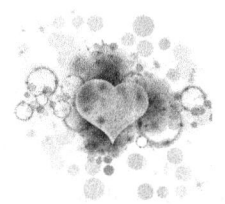

Introduction:

Losing Weight Is Easy

"In mythology, folklore and fantasy fiction, shapeshifting, or metamorphosis is the ability of an entity to physically transform into another being or form." (Wikipedia)

If there is one thing I am an expert at, it is how to shapeshift. Over the years friends have seen my body shift from size 26 to size 12 and back again—seemingly overnight. I've taken on several different forms, as you will see in photographs, and lost enough pounds over the years to equal ten of the woman writing this book.

Losing weight is easy. Finding the motivation to start—then keeping it off—that's challenging. Food has always been my easy-to-obtain, street-legal, drug of choice. One that is socially acceptable—until you eat yourself up to 300+ pounds and find yourself an outcast from "normal" society.

As I write these pages I believe I have undergone enough therapy and self-analysis to know my secret mental and emotional pitfalls. I don't know if writing about them will help you or if this will simply be another cathartic exercise. Either way, at least one of us will benefit by my doing so.

In these pages you will read about one woman's struggles ... and her triumphs. And you will find details from my current diary, pages from my calorie- and point-count log, menus and photographs of actual meals that I eat (many additional in full-color available on website to view and download in PDF format free of charge).

You will learn that I believe losing weight should be a creative, fun process filled with beautifully planned and presented meals. I use Crown Ming china and crystal even when I'm eating by myself—because I'm worth it.

I eat filling, balanced meals three times a day, including meats, snack primarily on fruit and have a special dessert, usually a rich cup of coffee and gourmet cookies, at night. In addition, I eat out with friends 2-4 times a week and never allow myself to feel deprived.

I vehemently oppose strenuous exercise because we usually set ourselves up for failure. I do incorporate at-work desk stretches and climbing stairs into my daily routine and do exercises my chiropractor has prescribed to strengthen core muscles.

My affirmation, in a picture frame in my bathroom, says:

I AM manifesting a body that is healthy, strong and pleasing to my eyes without consciously dieting or exercising.

Though my most successful weight loss efforts were supported by the Weight Watchers program, I found that it lacked the individualized personal attention I needed. I found Overeaters Anonymous which provided the personal attention with a sponsor, but it lacked the structure of Weight Watchers.

I realized that the times I had done best were when I followed Weight Watchers of the 1970s which limited us to one starchy item a day. How do I describe slicing one slice of bread into two melba thin slices and toasting them to make them sturdy enough to hold fillings?

Thus, this book explores my personal alchemy of combining weight loss plans and divinely inspired creative ideas, with an added measure of metaphysics, to help me become the best I am capable of being—physically, mentally, emotionally and spiritually.

Though not a "how-to" book, it details how I did it with enough information for you to replicate my results. I am a teacher, but you truly have your own answers. My job is to draw them out of you.

Namaskar,

Sharon

PART ONE

What Do You Have to Lose?

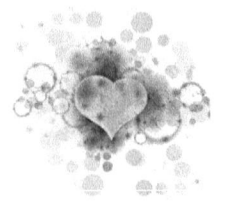

1: No More Playing Games

I remember the time I walked into a Rolls-Royce Owners Club party with my husband. Yes, I was an attractive, slender, well-dressed size 12, but that wasn't the reason heads turned. Members' reactions did not surprise me since the last time they had seen me I weighed 296 1/2-pounds and wore at least a size 22. Heads turned because they thought he had traded me in for a new model!

This same husband, after I lost weight, said that he knew women could gain weight. He had seen that happen many times. But once we had gained weight he didn't think it was possible for us to lose it. He started calling me his "trophy wife." I'm sure he meant it as a compliment. I, however, did not take it that way.

www.urbandictionary.com defines a "trophy wife" as "a young, attractive woman married to an older, more powerful man. His role in the relationship is to be her sugar daddy and provide her with power and material wealth." Considering that both of us worked 12 hours a day to build our business, I didn't consider that there was anything "trophy" about me!

I would have been so much happier if I could have just considered his words a compliment without worrying about what other people would think about me being a kept woman! Why couldn't I just focus on the "young, attractive" part?

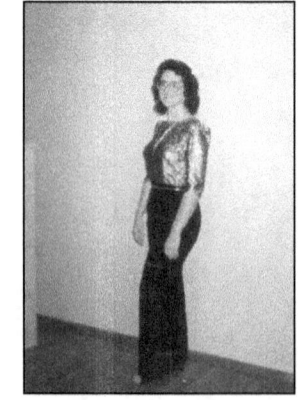

The summer of 1986, while a student in a community college (at age 36), I had lost 75-pounds and trained to be a Weight Watchers lecturer (see photo at right). Heads turned that time, too. Along with academic accolades for the first time in my life, I found myself the center of attention—and I liked that attention.

Fast forward to the present ... I am at an Inner Core group based on a book by the same title written by Rev. Robert L. Marshall of Unity Church in Orlando, Florida.

Members set intentions for exploring new frontiers in personal spiritual development and document examples in their lives. One of the participants talked about people with real or imagined illnesses using their stories to get attention.

You know the ones I'm talking about. A story comes to my mind of a woman who was in community college with me. After we graduated with our associate degrees we both went on to an upper level college. That college was about 1 1/2 hours from my home.

This classmate asked if she could carpool with me and offered to pay half the expenses. What could I say? Although I value my quiet downtime, and driving is relaxing for me, it made sense economically. So I said yes.

The minute she got in my car she started talking about her medical challenges. And she talked about them incessantly all the way to school ... and then all the way home. Having come from a childhood home in which I considered my mother to be a hypochondriac, I found the situation to be overwhelming .

I have laughingly said, in hindsight, that the worst part was that I couldn't get a word in edgewise to talk about my problems!

It got to a point that I felt I had no choice other than to tell her the truth about how her negativity and constant complaining was effecting me. It was disrupting the time I needed to think about my homework and to relax. So I confronted her.

Of course she got upset. And that was the last time I saw her.

But this story actually had, potentially, a happy ending. Six weeks later her husband called me. He said, "I don't know what you said to my wife, but whatever it was has made a tremendous difference in our home. She's a changed woman. Thank you."

I like to think that at the time, over 20 years before I became a Unity leader, that I already knew how to act in love rather than to react to my frustration (emotions).

Unfortunately, in the world we live in, most of these stories do not have that kind of ending. People who use illnesses in this manner are creating a escapist drama. I had been no different.

Suddenly my life flashed before me as I saw myself in an entirely new light. "That's me," I confessed to the group, "Only my addictive drama hinged on my weight going up and down." Either direction created drama that I could play off ... and I would milk it for all it was worth!

Just as suddenly, I understood that I didn't need it anymore.

My extreme focus on becoming a Licensed Unity Teacher (L.U.T.) under the auspices of Unity, while working full-time in the headquarters' Silent Unity Prayer Ministry, had earned me recognition at work, in my church, in groups in which I actively participate and among my friends.

I no longer needed the excess weight I was carrying and weight loss "insider tips," which are very much a part of who I am on a subconscious level, surfaced. This time, however, I only talked about changes in my body when I was asked ... and compliments/questions came frequently.

"How did you ...?"

"How do you ...?"

"Can you help me ...?"

I printed out sample pages of my daily log for friends. "These really helped me," they said. And I photographed actual meals and created pages from the photos. "Wow ... I love this! Thank you so much," they said. "How much do I owe you?" (See pages 170-211.)

So it seems that it is time to stop playing games and use the years of knowledge, and shapeshifting tricks that I've learned to help you lose weight—and show you how to have fun doing it.

Life is not meant to be stressful. I have learned to have fun, turn my job into fun, to enjoy all aspects of being human, and stress disappears. You can, too.

By now you are wondering what it means on the back cover when we say that "Sharon doesn't D-I-E-T—she plays with her food!"

No, I don't mean food fights. The idea of an apple whizzing by my head is not appealing ... or worse yet mashed potatoes! I could probably catch the apple.

I play with flavor combinations—spices, exotic sauces to tempt and satisfy the palate.

I play with colors and layout on a plate. Food tastes better, is more satisfying and you enjoy it even after the meal is finished if it tastes good and looks good.

I play with nutritional balances—fats, carbohydrates and proteins—for both nutrition and satiety level. It is kind of like balancing a checkbook. The more low point items you eat, the more quantity you can have, and the more satisfied you feel. Fruits and green vegetables are good examples.

Sharon Kay, M.A., L.U.T.

I play with budgeting in order to be a good steward of the money that the universe entrusts to me. In doing so I believe I benefit and the planet benefits by my use of less resources.

Although I understand that specialty food stores have some environmental advantages, I simply will not pay $1.00 for an "organic" orange when I can buy a regular orange for 25-cents especially considering that it is often impossible to prove "organic" unless you have a garden.

The most important alchemical ingredient you can use, and the most beneficial reaction you can elicit, comes from adding love to everything you eat. You'll learn why this is important when we discuss Dr. Masaru Emoto's studies of water crystals.

Eating balanced, economical meals is a science that I have been studying since the 1970s. At that time I was training to be a Weight Watcher's lecturer and actively involved in what was then called Home Demonstration Club (now County Extension Agency).

During that time of my life I did home canning and preserving for my family and for gift giving. I remember making a variety of types of pickles (dill, sweet, bread and butter) "scientifically" by using several different methods/recipes and taste testing them with friends.

I remember, too, making jalapeno jelly (Texas girl) to enhance meat dishes before it became readily available and popular in stores. I made my own rolls of refrigerator dough before you could buy them in the refrigerated section at stores and popped batch after batch into the oven for hot-out-of-the-oven cookies to serve guests.

Today I am a family of one. I entertain less, but I continue to be creative, packing as much flavor, quantity and nutrition as possible into low-calorie meals

I invite you to join me on this adventure in getting healthy.

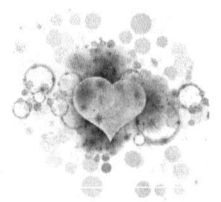

2: In the Flow of Normal

When I am in the flow of losing weight the word diet takes on an entirely different meaning. According to the *Merriam-Webster* online dictionary, a diet can be:

a: food and drink regularly provided or consumed
b: habitual nourishment
c: the kind and amount of food prescribed for a person or animal for a special reason
d: a regimen of eating and drinking sparingly so as to reduce one's weight (i.e. going on a diet)

When we say that we're "going on a diet," we usually think of it as "eating and drinking sparingly." Instead, I think in terms of "food and drink regularly provided or consumed." Instead of punishing myself, I am loving my body and providing nourishment that it needs and enjoys. I get into a flow of what I call "normal."

I like feeling normal.

I would define normal as people who eat what they want, when they want, and their bodies automatically self-regulate. One of the best things you can do for yourself is find a skinny friend to emulate. I know, I hear you saying, "But _____ eats anything s/he wants and never gains an ounce." If you have an opportunity to really observe that person, analyze their dietary/exercise habits.

Another option is to find a role model—someone you would like to emulate. It is important that their appearance and body build be in a range that would be realistic for you. In the 1970s, while learning Weight Watchers, I found my model—Wonder Woman!

Actually, it was Linda Carter, the woman behind the Wonder Woman costume. She was about my height, a body build and shape that I could realistically aspire to, and my hair at that time was long and dark brown. Look at the woman on page 2, including the thin gold belt (lariat) and see who you see now.

Sharon Kay, M.A., L.U.T.

Why did I choose Linda to be a role model? There was an article on the front page of a Weight Watchers magazine of that era telling how she had to lose 60-pounds before being chosen to play Wonder Woman. That gave me tremendous incentive to follow in her footsteps.

(**NOTE:** I know I'm not making this up, because it was a powerful incentive for me, but I cannot find corroborative documentation on the internet at this time. If any of you have a copy of that issue I would love to share it on the website.)

I have been married twice—to men whom I described as "skinny as a rail." The second marriage taught me a lot about how their minds/bodies work:

1) They did a lot more moving/strenuous work in the course of a normal day than I did sitting at a typewriter/computer;

2) When they ate, they might eat twice as much as I did, but they never ate in between meals and they never got up in the middle of the night to raid the refrigerator; and

3) If they gained 1-2 pounds, they felt it and cut back because they didn't feel good carrying extra pounds.

My second husband told me that there were two things he would not do if he didn't have to—eat and sleep. He considered both activities to be "fuel" for our bodies, not recreational drugs.

Imagine for a moment filling your car with gasoline. If it has a 20-gallon tank, you simply cannot force 21 gallons into it. In fact, even after a light goes on warning you that you need fuel, it will usually hold less than 20 gallons. If you try to force more in what happens?

Now translate that into your body. How many times have I force-fed 30-40 gallons into my frame that was only intended to hold 20 gallons.

In other words, charts say I should weigh about 175-pounds. If I continually feed my body the calories that would be required by a 300-pound individual, what do you think is going to happen?

Yes! I am going to become the size my intake is designed to maintain. If I eat 3,000 calories a day when my body only needs 1,200 there is no way that I am going to be able to make myself do enough exercise to offset the extra 1,800 calories.

A friend asked me tonight how I was feeling. She was concerned. "You are looking great ... but how are you really feeling?" She's been on enough diets to know that most weight loss programs that show the immediate results I am demonstrating leave you feeling weak and even depressed.

"I'm feeling fine," I said, not convinced she believed me. As you probably know there are hundreds, perhaps thousands, of diets being recommended by people who are considered experts in the field. Many promise you 30-40-pound losses quickly.

Effective, long-lasting weight loss does not involve fad diets, taking pills, fasting, extreme exercise, special (costly) foods or programs. It simply takes foods that can be found in any store and reframes the way we look at them. It takes foods we already like and uses simple management tools to control the number of calories instead of letting them control us.

In my opinion, any diet that asks you to vary dramatically from your normal way of eating is setting you up for failure. I guarantee that if you have to force yourself to eat or drink things you don't like to lose weight, you will not stick to them long-term. And, when you return to your regular eating habits, you will gain those pounds back quickly; thus setting yourself up for what is called "yo-yo" dieting.

Yes, if you do what I did, you will have to give up things like donuts and fried chicken, except on very special occasions, but you will eat real food, things you actually like, and not feel deprived. In other words, you will learn how to manage your diet rather than allowing emotions to control what you put in your mouth.

One of my long-time friends tells people that if I had $1,000 and she had $2,000 she would run out before I did. It is true. You've heard the phrase "pinch a penny until it squeals". I can do the same thing with a calorie.

What do I mean by that? One of the best examples I can give is potatoes. You can choose one ounce of potato chips, which have absolutely no nutritional value, for 150 calories—or you can have a whole medium size baked potato, loaded with nutrients, with butter flavored spray and spices, for about the same number of calories.

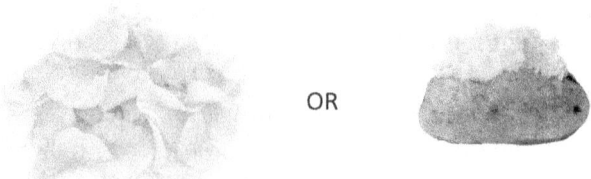

OR

Potato chips are lightweight, loaded with oil they soaked up and salty. One of the best marketing slogans ever created was, "Bet you can't eat just one!" Truthfully, how many of us can eat just one ounce? And then an hour later you are hungry again.

Sharon Kay, M.A., L.U.T.

A key to successful weight loss is feeling full when you eat and the only way to do that is by making the choice to consume primarily items that are high in nutritional value, high in satiety quotient and low in calories. Most sweet or salty foods meet none of those criteria.

My favorite mother-in-law once said about Weight Watchers, "I've figured out how you lose weight. It's from carrying all that food around." For those of you not familiar with the Weight Watchers program, the plan allows you to eat LARGE quantities of low calorie, high nutrition foods such as fruits, vegetables and lean meat.

Thus, not only did I bring things I could eat in liberal quantities to family get-togethers, I also ate large quantities of foods that were 0-points on my program,

The truth is that not all calories are created equal and successful weight loss is about learning how to balance them.

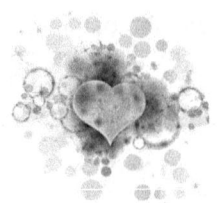

3: Fuel for Our Bodies

Yes, a calorie is a calorie is a calorie, but it takes:

9 calories to equal 1 gram of fat
7 calories to equal 1 gram of alcohol
4 calories to equal 1 gram of protein or carbohydrate

Which do you think you should eat more of? Protein and carbohydrates seem logical, right? But protein and carbohydrate grams are not created equal.

Protein is fairly easy to explain in a non-technical way, because it is simply the ratio of fat to protein found in various meats. For example, I go to the deli department in my grocery store and buy thick slices (1/2" to 3/4") of 98% fat-free meats for lunches and dinners. I like bacon for breakfast 2-3 times per week, plus bacon, tomato and lettuce sandwiches occasionally, and choose precooked bacon which heats in 30 seconds in a microwave, is crispy, tastes like regular bacon—and most of the fat has been pressed out!

You will, however, hear people talking about "good" proteins and "bad" proteins. I can agree that some proteins such as fish and chicken, and organic free-range buzzwords, may be better for the environment. And lean as opposed to fatty meats may be better for our bodies. But there are times in our life when we may not be financially able to buy the best quality, environmentally and body-friendly choices. And, while beans and rice are very good for you as a complete protein, a diet of nothing but beans and rice can get very monotonous.

My diet approach, as discussed in this book, focuses on a balanced variety of proteins, carbohydrates and fats. I often take inexpensive processed protein and pasta TV dinners and fortify them with fresh vegetables and fruit. (See page 158 on "Dressing Up TV Dinners.")

Carbohydrates are more complicated. Just as with protein, you may have heard that there are "good" carbs and "bad" carbs. I don't like to put anything in a "bad" category, but some carbs are handled more efficiently by our bodies.

Sharon Kay, M.A., L.U.T.

The easiest way to describe the difference is by using the Glycemic Index. According to www.bodybuilding.com, "Carbohydrates that break down slowly, releasing glucose gradually into the blood stream, have a low glycemic index. A lower glycemic index suggests slower rates of digestion and absorption of the sugars and starches in the foods and may also indicate greater extraction from the liver and periphery of the products of carbohydrate digestion."

What does that translate to for you and me? Carbohydrates in a baked potato, without added fat, break down more slowly than carbs in a donut and have less calories, We feel more satisfied while eating the potato, thus we do not get hungry as soon. I eat a lot of potatoes, white as well as yams, without feeling guilt afterward.

In addition, I eat as much fruit as I want without guilt. Originally it was because Weight Watchers teaches that we don't have to count points for fruit. But I have diabetic friends whose doctors restrict the amount of fruit they can eat. So I wasn't sure what to tell them in relation to losing weight the way I propose.

A friend recently shared a web link about Dr. Michael Gregor who reports on studies showing that people in control groups who ate up to 20 pieces of fruit a day (!) did not have significant increases in blood sugar levels. The article in its entirety can be found at:

http://www.forksoverknives.com/is-it-possible-to-eat-too-much-fruit/

A summary by Naomi Imatome-Yun, managing editor of *Forks Over Knives* magazine, says that,

"New, emerging literature has shown that low-dose fructose from whole, natural foods may actually benefit blood sugar control. So having a piece of fruit with each meal could lower, not raise the blood sugar response. But what about fructose toxicity? The threshold for toxicity of fructose may be around 50 grams. The problem is, that that's how much fructose the average adult consumes in one day. That means that half of all adults are likely above the threshold for fructose toxicity, and adolescents currently average 75 grams.

"Is that the limit for added sugars or for all fructose? If we don't want more than 50 grams and there's about ten grams in a piece of fruit, should we limit our fruit consumption to five pieces a day? According to the Harvard Health Letter: 'The nutritional problems of fructose and sugar come when they are added to foods. Fruit, on the other hand, is beneficial in almost any amount.'

"What do they mean almost? Can we eat ten fruits a day? How about twenty?

"We don't have to guess. Its actually been put to the test. In one study, seventeen people were made to eat 20 servings a day of fruit. Despite the extraordinarily high fructose content of this diet (about 200 grams per day, or the amount in 8 cans of soda), the investigators reported no adverse effects (and possible benefit actually) for body weight, blood pressure, insulin, and lipid levels after three to six months.

"More recently, Jenkins and colleagues put people on a 20 servings of fruit a day diet for a few weeks with no adverse effects on weight, blood pressure, or triglycerides and an astounding 38 point drop in LDL cholesterol.

"There was one side effect, though. Their bathroom habits became very regular."

So ... throw away the Ex-Lax and eat more fresh whole fruit. "Fresh" and "whole" are the key words. We need to chew on the actual fruit in order to feel satisfied as opposed to juicing them or put them into a blender and drinking them. It is amazing how many calories you can drink!

In regard to fats, you will read elsewhere that I have gotten rid of butter and margarine in my home and use primarily coconut oil for cooking because I am thoroughly convinced of its benefits both internally and externally.

According to www.WebMD.com:

"Coconut oil is used for diabetes, heart disease, chronic fatigue, Crohn's disease, irritable bowel syndrome (IBS), Alzheimer's disease, thyroid conditions, energy, and boosting the immune system. Ironically, despite coconut oil's high calorie and saturated fat content, some people use it to lose weight and lower cholesterol.

"Coconut oil is sometimes applied to the skin as a moisturizer and to treat a skin condition called psoriasis."

I don't compulsively avoid other fats when eating out, but it is the only oil I keep in my home. If I'm going to "spend" nine calories on one gram of oil, I want it to be the best possible value for my food budget. I try to consume two teaspoons a day, plus I use it externally for things as widely disparate as hand cream and personal lubricant.

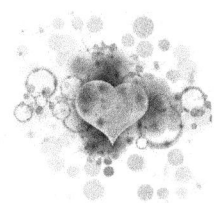

4: How to Decide What Plan

Questions I would ask in deciding what weight loss program to use are:

1. Is it something I can live with long-term?
2. Do I like the things I will be allowed to eat?
3. How difficult will it be for me to prepare the meals?
4. How fast do they predict that I will lose a substantial amount of weight?
5. Has any plan worked for me in the past?

The first three are about personal preferences. Number four is critical. If you are being promised that you can lose a lot of weight quickly the plan is NOT, in my opinion, a healthy option.

Five is probably the most reliable indicator of success, but if you found that you didn't stick to it, as was true for me with Weight Watchers, you may find that you have to combine the principles of that plan with other methods.

Counting calories is still a very viable weight loss plan and is what I recommend if you don't already have a plan that you know works for you when you actually follow it. Counting calories costs almost nothing to implement and there are tools on the Internet to help you figure out how many calories you can eat in a day and lose weight.

It is, however, critical that you learn proper nutrition. My beloved mother-in-law, when told by her doctor to eat more vegetables, went home to corn and potatoes. While I recommend these vegetables over grains such as breads (wheat) and rice (see Food Pyramid on page 16), they count as starches—not vegetables. You can learn what a balanced diet consists of through websites, books or by scheduling an appointment with a nutritionist. I also have a section on my website called "Balanced Nutrition."

We are programmed by our culture to believe that the bigger, the more expensive something is, the better. But there is a subculture promoting going back to the simple life. While I am not ready to give up my cell phone, laptop, etc., there really are some things that can stand to be revived—such as pushing ourselves away from the table when we've consumed the number of calories our bodies need for nutrition.

On www.caloriecount.com we read that, "In order to lose weight, you need your calorie intake to be less than your total daily calories burned. Using our weight loss calculator, you'll arrive at the calories you need to eat to reach your goal weight. Remember, there's a healthy range in which to achieve this loss. Restricting too much can be harmful to your health. The goal is to reach a weight loss of about 0.5-2 pounds per week so that your body has time to adjust and you are more likely to keep the weight off in the long-term."

The first page at www.caloriecount.com/tools/calories-goal asked me for my current weight and my goal weight. The second page asked my gender, weight, height and activity level.

The results I got said that I "... should consume about 1,249 calories a day to reach your goal weight ... this is at a reasonable weight loss average of 1.5 pounds per week." As you will find further into the book, this is very close to what I am doing.

the website includes a valid warning that women should eat no less than 1,200 calories a day and a man no less than 1,500. It also reminds us that the sexes were not created equal from the beginning! (laughter) A man's metabolism, as a rule, burns more calories even at rest than a woman's.

This is just one of many websites yielded from asking the question, "How many calories can I eat and still lose weight?" Play around with different websites and find one that is free to use and has tools you can use to plan nutritionally balanced meals. This one is free.

If, however, you do not have a computer, you can simply photocopy page __ in this book and manually enter what you eat and do the math—it's not rocket science. Or you can even use an old blank check ledger.

Instead of playing games with carbs and fats, consider that no one food is "bad." Moderation is the key and is easily controlled. We can consume too much of anything. I see a coworker carrying a gallon jug of water to work every day. Can we drink too much water? According to the Mayo Clinic, yes it is possible:

"Although uncommon, it is possible to drink too much water. When your kidneys are unable to excrete the excess water, the electrolyte (mineral) content of the blood is diluted, resulting in low sodium levels in the blood, a condition called hyponatremia. Endurance athletes, such as marathon runners who drink large amounts of water, are at higher risk of hyponatremia. In general, though, drinking too much water is rare in healthy adults who eat an average American diet."

The article goes on to say that, "You don't need to rely only on what you drink to meet your fluid needs. What you eat also provides a significant portion of your fluid needs. On average, food provides about 20 percent of total water intake. For example, many fruits and vegetables, such as watermelon and spinach, are 90 percent or more water by weight."

In regard to keeping life simple, there are few foods easier to prepare and eat than fresh fruit.

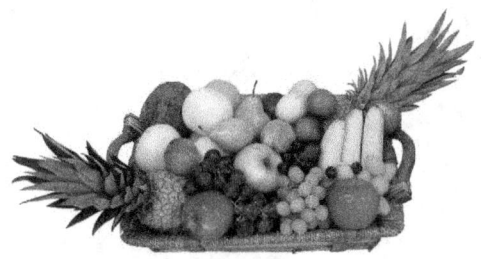

Food Pyramids

I did quite a lot of research to find a food pyramid that accurately reflected my concept of how to provide adequate nutrition to our bodies and at the same time lose weight.

If you do an Internet search for "Food Pyramid" you will have dozens of choices. None of them, in my opinion, reflect a style of eating that most of us could follow for a extended period of time.

It got to a point that I decided to create my own pyramid which you will find on the next page A larger full-color version of this pyramid can be found on my website at www.SharonKays.website/tools/ pyramid. And you may want to use my *Shape Shifter's Coloring Book for Adults, Tens & Kids* as a learning tool.

Shape Shifter's Food Pyramid

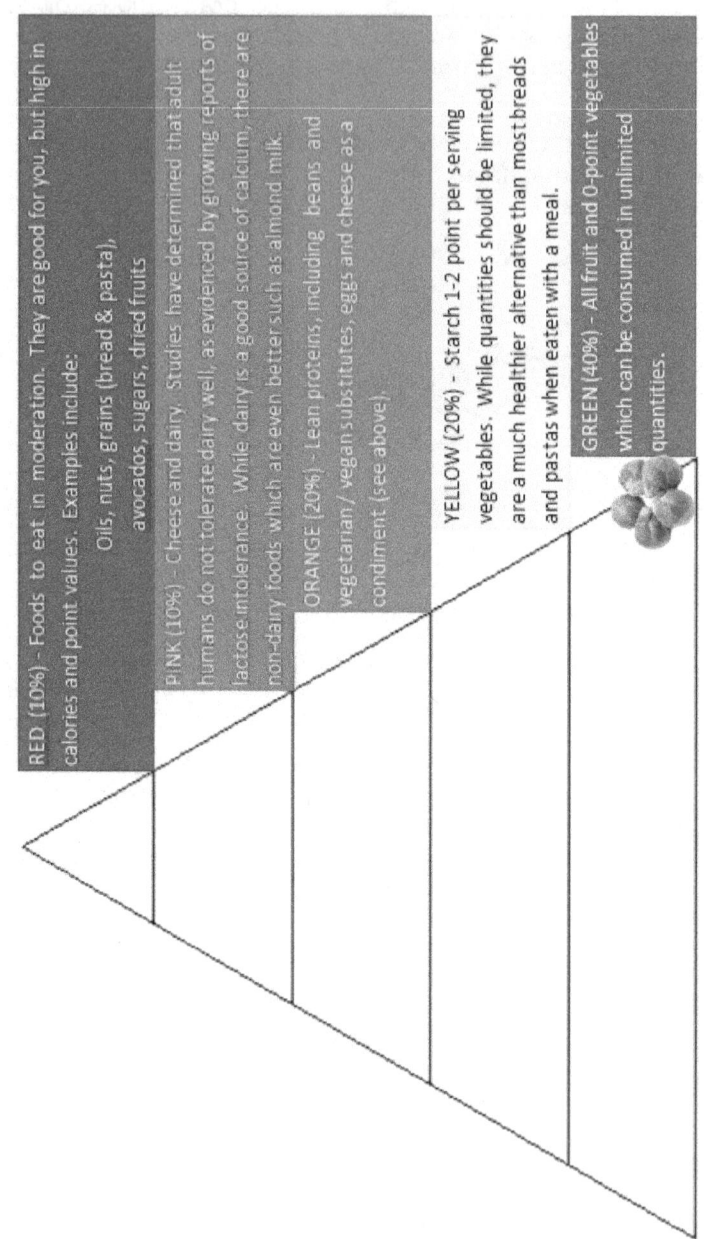

RED (10%) - Foods to eat in moderation. They are good for you, but high in calories and point values. Examples include:

Oils, nuts, grains (bread & pasta), avocados, sugars, dried fruits

PINK (10%) - Cheese and dairy. Studies have determined that adult humans do not tolerate dairy well, as evidenced by growing reports of lactose intolerance. While dairy is a good source of calcium, there are non-dairy foods which are even better such as almond milk.

ORANGE (20%) - Lean proteins, including beans and vegetarian / vegan substitutes, eggs and cheese as a condiment (see above).

YELLOW (20%) - Starch 1-2 point per serving vegetables. While quantities should be limited, they are a much healthier alternative than most breads and pastas when eaten with a meal.

GREEN (40%) - All fruit and 0-point vegetables which can be consumed in unlimited quantities.

EXAMPLE: I love brussels sprouts so I copied and pasted a small image of this 0-point vegetable onto the pyramid.

Sharon Kay, M.A., L.U.T.

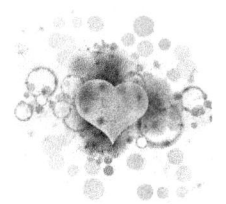

5: One Plan, Multiple Resources

Part One discussed aspects of the games that we play with our weight, what eating normal looks like to me, food as fuel for our bodies, and how to decide what plan will work best for us. We are physical, mental, emotional and spiritual beings; therefore, I have attempted to divide these aspects of our being into the next five parts, including our environment. There is a lot of overlap. Roughly the parts cover:

Mental Issues—Things we consciously think about that challenge our ability to lose weight.

Emotional Issues—Deeply ingrained subconscious factors from family, friends and society which work in our subconscious to undermine conscious efforts to lose weight.

Physical Issues—Things that have to do with our bodies (i.e. health, finances).

Spiritual Issues—Metaphysical aspects of our personalities.

Environmental Issues—Factors in our home and relationships that play a significant role in whether or not we succeed.

One size does NOT fit all in clothes, nor does any one weight loss program work for everyone. My combination is:

Weight Watchers	Counting calories
Overeaters Anonymous	Sceniuses
Church groups	Workplace

These groups have all played a role in making me the woman I am today. There is some truth in, "It is not my fault ... you made me ..." If people around us praise us, give us positive feedback, we as humans have a tendency to want to do more of whatever behavior earned the acclaim. And, of course, the reverse is also true. We avoid painful experiences and often that means hiding behind fat.

Our primary job in life is to surround ourselves with people and things that make us feel good about ourselves. I found my nirvana at Unity Village, Missouri. Friends who love the beach are in heaven in Galveston, Texas.

Yet it is seldom the geography that draws us. There is a much deeper level by which we are attracted to places and people. Throughout the pages of this book you will find ways to grow in all areas, on all levels—all of which play roles in your perception of yourself and thereby contribute to your body size.

I create you in my image of what I expect you to be ... and you create me in your image of what you expect me to be. In fact, and this is mind-expanding if you don't understand the concept, we create "God" in our own image. This is easily illustrated by putting a group of people around a table and asking them to describe God. If you have ten people, you will get ten different answers—even if all are members of the same church.

Personally, I am ready for you to begin creating me in your image of a tall, vivacious, slender woman with unlimited potential and bestselling books that bless everyone who reads them. ☺

Unfortunately, not everything is either black or white. Many of our issues are varying shades of gray. Something that may be causing us enough pain to raid the cookie jar may come disguised as a pleasant memory.

The next two sections discuss mental and emotional issues that I had to recognize and deal with.

Sharon Kay, M.A., L.U.T.

After reading this section I realized that I _____

_____

_____

_____

_____

_____

_____

_____

_____

_____

_____

_____

_____

_____

_____

_____

_____

_____

_____

_____

_____

_____

_____

Sharon Kay, M.A., L.U.T.

PART TWO

What Are

Your

Mental Issues?

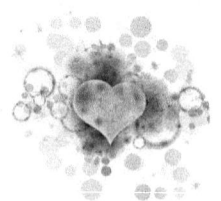

6: The Alchemy of Thoughts and Emotions

This section is all about me. It is not specific to you, though you may recognize some things from your life in my dramas. If you are reading this book, we probably have a lot of similarities.

In the process of figuring out who I am and why I have been overweight most of my life, I did a lot of soul searching and analysis. For me, being overweight began as a child, and you will read things from my past about family members.

I don't say any of this to blame or demean anyone whom I have chosen to play roles in my life. (Yes, I believe we are even attracted to our parents before we are born.) Rather, I use stories and examples to illustrate factors that played a role in making me who I am today.

Food as a Reward

One scenario that I remember from childhood involves a step-grandmother who did not like my biological grandmother—and took every opportunity to let me know it—but who nevertheless did things like teaching me how to crochet (for which I am very grateful).

An unfortunate aspect of crocheting for me was rewarding myself for a job well done. I remember in vivid detail sitting on the sofa crocheting (painstakingly, with tiny thread and tiny needle, not the yarn most of us use today). As I finished each round, a cookie, or whatever my indulgence was that day, was my reward for doing a good job.

Crochet another round, reward ... crochet ... reward ... crochet ... reward.

To this day rewards usually come in the form of food for me.

　　　　　　　　　　　Sharon Kay, M.A., L.U.T.

Intelligence vs. Beauty

I grew up being taught to believe that brains were more important than looks. This was reinforced in my church where I learned that thinking yourself pretty was vanity. There are plenty of scriptures in the Bible to back that up! So all the time I was growing up, and it carried on throughout the majority of my life, I saw myself as intelligent, but fat and unattractive.

At that time, this was a highly emphasized moral value for young women in my church. It was, we were told, the gorgeous cheerleaders, the girls who got all the boys—who also got pregnant and, ultimately, were ostracized by the society that created them.

Along those same lines, I envied people with musical abilities. Having been kicked out of a teen church choir for "not being able to carry a tune in a paper sack," I assumed that it was a pretty safe bet that I had no musical talent. So I focused on "playing" the keys of a typewriter which I was very good at. Years later someone said to me, "You have fingers that were made to either play the piano or type." Funny ... no one ever mentioned, and I didn't figure it out, that I could have done both.

Knowing what I know now from metaphysical teachings, it is no wonder that I created a body of a fat woman who sat at a desk all day. Actually, there seemed to me to be no other option. As a slender, high energy woman (on the occasions I lost weight), I created nothing but problems for myself. Of course it wasn't really me creating them, it was societal expectations and norms. But I didn't understand that.

Low Self-Esteem

When I was 17, and pleasingly plump, I met a 24-year-old man and fell in love. (Is any 17-year-old capable of knowing what love is?) In actuality, I was escaping my childhood home and, in retrospect, realize that I felt he was the best match I would ever be able to make. That was a downright shame, because I had earned the award for the most outstanding business student in my high school, was offered and accepted a job with a major company in the town and, when I look at my wedding photographs, I was a gorgeous brunette with long wavy hair. But I couldn't see or value those truths.

We spent 22 years of marriage putting each other down. When the first song you dance to, and call "our song," is "Please Release Me" by Elvis Presley, is it any wonder the marriage didn't last? I remember so well our "teasing" one another by asking, "Why did you marry me?" Reply: "Because no one else would have you."

At the time these things were being bandied around the table, I remember a friend's husband playing footsies under the table—and, unfortunately, I also remember being sorely tempted to take him up on it. I didn't … but I got the name without playing the game when I apologized to his wife—for my thoughts.

I remember, too, the Baptist minister who was my husband's fishing buddy. I wasn't interested in this one, but when my husband was told that his friend had made a pass at me, guess who was blamed for "tempting" his friend?

Words are incredibly powerful. Combine them with emotions, negative or positive, and they can be devastating.

For example, if someone is hit with a 2" x 4" stud board and their arm is broken, how long will it take to heal? According to the Internet, it will take approximately six weeks. If someone is hit with words such as "I hate you, you are fat and ugly, you are stupid," how long will it take to heal? They may never heal. Though I believe I have healed through the power of forgiveness, I can still remember childhood taunts of "Fatty, fatty, 2" x 4", can't get through the kitchen door."

On the other hand, positive words create positive results.

Rejection

At the end of 20 years of marriage, I learned that I had spent a woman's most sexually active years with a pedophile who had rejected me after we had two children. Is it any wonder that I turned to food to stuff my emotions ... mostly in bed, at night, alone? The only regret I have about divorcing is that I didn't do it sooner and save my children some grief.

I do not believe that all marital problems can be resolved amicably. Nor do I believe that all marriages are ordained by God even when the marriage takes place in a church.

You may remember that I had lost 75-pounds during that marriage. After the divorce I gained it and more back.

Was it Weight Watchers fault that I didn't keep the weight off? No. Weight Watchers is a great program and, if you have never been to one of their meetings or learned the program, I strongly encourage you to do so. This book and my counseling are supplemental material. They are the added motivation that most of us need.

I remember so well the games that many of us, myself included, played while following Weight Watchers' program. If you weighed on a Wednesday night, it was okay to indulge in treats and foods that were not allowed on the program for 2-3 days. It got to be a game to see how much you could eat and still lose weight at your next weigh-in.

Obviously, if we had followed the program seven days a week instead of four-and-a-half we would have lost weight faster, gotten the program into our subconscious, and have had a better chance of keeping it off. Some did, but my experience is that they were the rare exceptions.

Weight Watchers, in my opinion, is the most sensible, healthy weight loss program around, and it is highly modifiable. The only problem I have with today's program is that it tries to please all of the people all of the time and that's just not possible. Grossly overweight people need more structure.

In regard to Weight Watchers, it was more about me rejecting them than the program not being good for me. I am very grateful for all that I learned through the program. Could I have learned it in other ways? Yes. But it was my path at the time.

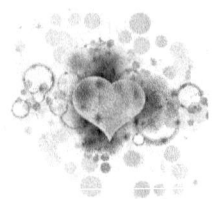

7: The Science Behind Our Thoughts and Emotions

A scientific approach to studying effects of thoughts on water came to my attention several years ago. Dr. Masaru Emoto of Japan took samples of water, put drops in test tubes, taped emotional words and phrases to tubes such as "I love you," "peace," "hate," "I'm going to kill you." He then photographed frozen samples under a microscope and documented results in several books titled *Hidden Messages in Water,* Vols. 1, 2, 3 and 4.

Water that "felt" loved, or any other positive emotion, formed beautiful crystal, snowflake-like structures. Water that felt hatred or any negative emotion formed a turbulent structure. I considered what this might mean in regard to water going into my body, knowing that our bodies are 75-80% water—and immediately understood why we have been told for years to bless our food and drink before eating!

Women in India are trained from childhood to put love into their cooking. During two trips to India I had the privilege of learning from my hostess. Whole spices are ground for seasoning and love is poured into those spices. Additional love is added in every step of the meal from dal (lentils or peas) to naan (bread). What were *we* taught? Fast food restaurants? Frozen TV dinners? Eating in a car in our misguided struggles to be "Supermoms." It wasn't love that we were pouring into our meals, but rather frustration over never feeling good enough.

How did/do we treat ourselves? Consider what effects we may be having on our bodies when we curse certain parts with words such as "thunder thighs," "You are so fat!" "What man/woman would ever want you?" Based on Dr. Emoto's results, and Unity teachings, is it any wonder that we get exactly what we perceive—beautiful, light energy bodies or dense globs of negative energy.

Yet so many of us go around in a constant state of denial. How many times have I laid the blame on a washing machine for shrinking my slacks ... when in reality it was my body that had expanded. This refusal to face reality constitutes psychological *denial.*

On the other hand, I learned through metaphysical studies that using "denials" as a way to heal our emotions works. A spiritual denial is simply a statement, of preferably 10 words or less, denying that something has power over you. For example, I might say that, "Food has no control over my emotions."

Our spiritual nature abhors a vacuum. In other words, if we throw out the trash with a denial we have to fill the empty container (our conscious) with something positive and affirming. So we then affirm, "I am choosing nutritious food that blesses my body."

Why does this work? It reprograms our mental, emotional and spiritual circuitry. I liken the brain to a processing plant. What we put into it goes through a process akin to alchemy and transforms our thoughts. If we add the emotion of love in talking to our bodies, the re-action is like Dr. Emoto's ice crystals—we become beautiful inside, and it reflects outwardly, regardless our physical attributes. What I call our Christ light, a spark of divinity within each person, shines more brightly.

A Course in Miracles teaches that there are only two emotions: fear and love. Consider the following table:

FEAR-BASED	LOVE-BASED
Anger	Beauty
Hate	Passion
Distrust	Compassion
Jealousy	Trust

If we express disgust at our bodies, we do so out of fear—fear that we are not desirable enough to attract a partner, fear that we will never be good enough in the workplace to compete with coworkers for the best jobs, fear of being a failure.

On the flip side of the coin, I made a decision to love my body, just as it is (at any point in time), and I invite you to do the same. Some days I may like it better than other days, but choosing not to love it is no longer an option.

Sciences of physical, mental, emotional and spiritual arenas are merging into a blended science which recognizes that we are so much more than our bodies. Quantum physics has demonstrated that we have control over our environment without ever touching it by the thoughts that we think.

Through our thoughts, we control the way our bodies look and act. Forget the negative things other people say (including, perhaps especially, doctors). Their words have no control over us—unless we believe them.

Our own thoughts, just like thoughts sent to water, are extremely powerful. They define whether you are a pauper or a prince; a bag lady or an executive. Although there are instances of brain damage and mental illnesses that render people incapable of controlling their thoughts, a vast majority of us have this ability.

Unfortunately, many choose not to exercise this tool. We have become so accustomed to allowing other people to tell us how to think that we have forgotten how to think for ourselves. "But," you say, "I don't listen to other people. Most of them are a bunch of idiots."

What about those magazines you read? The movies you watch? The music you listen to? These are experts, aren't they? They're successful ... so they must know what they're talking about. You listen and you do what they tell you to do. As a society, we are brainwashed. We run to the store to buy the latest convenience or high priced, high calorie fast foods advertised.

And the best example yet ... you are reading this book. You see my before and after photographs on pages 95 and 98. You may have seen me in person and heard me talk. So I'm an expert, aren't I? I obviously know what I'm doing when I talk about how to lose weight.

Well, guess what, honey (my Texas diner talk). It is late Monday night as I write this and I've been on a binge since Saturday and am praying that I can get my act together so that the scales weigh less next Saturday morning than they did last Saturday.

It started Saturday evening when a girlfriend and I went to California Pizza Kitchen. I looked at menus before going. It was my choice to go there. It's not the best choice, but I figured I could handle it reasonably well ... after all, I know what I'm doing.

I ordered a Fire Roasted Chili Relleno stuffed with chicken, cheese, roasted corn and black bean salsa, wild mushrooms, spinach, eggplant, cilantro and avocado salsa verde from the "Light Adventures" menu at 420 calories. Good choice! I was going to have a cup of soup with it, but my girlfriend wanted a Shaved Mushroom and Spinach Flatbread. I offered to split one with her. She wanted a whole one. "The crust is really thin—so that doesn't count, does it?" She grinned. So we each ordered one (400 calories).

And, yes, we would have the sourdough bread with olive oil freebies (2 tablespoons olive oil equals 240 calories plus the bread chunks [small]).

And I suggested we top it off by splitting a tiramisu. On this she agreed to one-half—410 calories **per person**!

Total calories—over 1500.

Yes, I justified, even with this splurge, it is not a problem. I've eaten about what I would eat if I were on maintenance and there are six days left in the week.

Sunday—Easter Sunday! I worked at my job that day; then went to an afternoon church service where I also work as a volunteer. And I nibbled whenever and wherever something was available.

Monday ... I don't want to talk about it other than to say that I am sitting here feeling miserable. Yet, if you saw me three days ago, then again today, I wouldn't look any different to you. The difference is in how I feel about myself and right now it is easy to tell myself that I'm only human, but I really want to do what is best for me—and be an example for you.

You get the picture, though. We really are like alcoholics. Betcha can't eat just one. The real problem with going off my abstinence program is how hard it is to get back on track. Overeaters Anonymous (OA) defines "abstinence" as developing a plan that works for you and sticking to it.

For more on creating a plan and sticking to it you may want to read the book *Abstinence*, a combination of motivational articles written by OA members and published by OA. The copy I first used was a 2001 edition, but there are other editions, each with different stories.

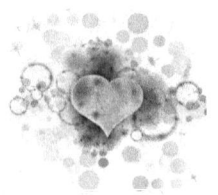

8: Mental and Emotional Challenges

In the late 1970s, while a member of Weight Watchers for the first time, I met a fellow member whom I considered to be gorgeous. (She became a well-known writer of romantic fiction.) I had lost most of my weight (see page 2) and she said to me, "Go home, clean out your clothes closet, and throw away anything that doesn't make heads turn when you walk in the door."

My self-esteem, my healthy ego, were almost non-existent at the time. I could not understand what a tremendous compliment she was paying me; that she was telling me I was gorgeous. In retrospect, Unity teaches that what we see in others is also true of us I could see it in her, but at that time I could not accept beauty as being a good thing—and who I am, as well.

Psychologists say that it takes five years after losing weight for a person to be able to look in the mirror and actually see the person they have become. Mental and emotional challenges to losing weight not only surround us via societal input, but they are deep-seated, in-grained thoughts and feelings indoctrinated since birth that we have to recognize and erase from our subconscious before we can truly appreciate our new bodies.

I realized that my weight was a desperate, albeit ridiculous, attempt at hiding. So I first had to figure out why I would exercise so much discipline, implement dramatic organizational abilities, etc., to lose weight—then gain it all back. It didn't make sense for an otherwise intelligent woman to apparently sabotage her efforts.

Weight is a wall we put up to protect ourselves from being hurt. Unfortunately, it is a self-destructive wall in that the pain we try to escape is amplified by the excess weight and hurtful things that other people say and do based on their first impressions of us as "fat."

According a June 2003 article by the National Geographic Society "... more than 160 million people in India are considered 'Untouchable'—people tainted by their birth into a caste system that deems them impure, less than human. Human rights abuses against these people, known as Dalits, are legion." This is in spite of the fact that in 1950 the practice was made illegal by law.

According to a June 2013 article by the National Center for Bio-technical Information, a branch of the National Institutes of Health, **"Adjusting for self-report biases, we estimate that in 2010 15.5 million adult Americans or 6.6% of the population had an actual BMI >40 kg m(-2). The prevalence of clinically severe obesity continues to be increasing, although less rapidly in more recent years than prior to 2005."**

Does America have its own group of Untouchables today?

I am listening to a woman who wants to talk about her son. She tells me that he is a business man, a husband and father. It had been over two years since she had seen him and he and his family had just left.

She spat the next words out:

"He was FAT the last time I saw him. Now he's OBESE! It makes me sick to look at him!"

Her attempt to disguise her disgust was buried in "concern for his health."

Yes, this man probably does have health challenges ... but her antipathy/callousness will kill her just as surely being overweight will kill him.

Though employers are not by law allowed to discriminate on the bases of race, color, religion, national origin or sex, no such law exists for hiring a man or woman who is considered obese in an employer's opinion.

Many other situations could be cited, but, as a religious leader one of my most challenging observations is how few churches make accommodations for people with extra girth. Do large people not need spirituality as much as a slender person?

When I see a grossly overweight person riding in a motorized shopping cart at a grocery store I want so badly to go up to them and say, as Jesus the Christ did, "Rise and be healed." A minority of those individuals do have medical challenges that require use of a cart, but a vast majority simply need to lose weight. If you look at my before picture on page 112, I am living proof that it can be done.

But we force ourselves to go on diets that don't work—the cabbage soup diet, liquid protein, protein shakes, fasts, pre-packaged meals that eliminate our need to make choices, etc.

Everything we try ultimately results in failure because we're looking for a magic potion. We have not learned to take responsibility for our own actions. We have not learned how to love our bodies just as they are and treat them with the respect they deserve.

I cannot bear to watch morbidly obese people on shows like *The Biggest Loser* being humiliated in the guise of "helping" them lose weight. Losing weight quickly, under extremely stressful situations, pretty much guarantees that the person will end up worse than when they started. Cruel, inhumane treatment under any guise is still abuse no matter how much a person may be paid, or stand to win in a weight loss contest, to endure it.

The Huffington Post, on February 27, 2014, ran an article on contestants' lives after the show. The article reads:

"It's no secret that "The Biggest Loser" is unhealthy. Outlets like The New York Times itemized the hazardous medical implications of such extreme and rapid weight loss as early as 2009. Yet, the 'Biggest Loser' is flawed beyond the questionable practice of more than six hours of exercise a day. Ultimately, the concept of diets—absurdly rigorous or not—are faulty attempts at healthy living. And the imposition of such an intense weight adjustment has an alarming impact once the cast leaves the ranch.

"Huff Post TV spoke to past contestants to see what the real world was like after "The Biggest Loser," and the techniques they used to keep (or attempt to keep) the weight off. Despite the intensity of the experience on campus, often returning to the real world was a more rigorous task.

"After Rachel Frederickson's controversial win at the end of this most current season, health concerns relating to the show resurfaced with greater force than ever before. While these issues are valid, the most crucial failing of the show is its unrealistic expectations about life after the ranch and the relative abandonment of contestants once the finale has aired."

For the full article go to:

http://www.huffingtonpost.com/2014/02/27/biggest-loser_n_4868870.html.

You will hear me say over and over again that healthy weight loss does not come from an overnight magic potion. It takes motivation, dedication and discipline. But I can tell you that it is worth it.

Possibly the best thing my first husband did for me was to encourage me to not start smoking. I began my working career straight out of high school at age 16 in an era when cigarette companies had

Sharon Kay, M.A., L.U.T.

people stationed in major businesses giving out free samples. I recall little packages of five cigarettes—but a pretty girl could go by as many times as she wanted.

I would smoke a cigarette on the way home from work (and believed I was hiding it from my mother!). After we started dating, my future husband said, "I don't have a right to tell you not to smoke ... but I can tell you how hard it is to quit. I wish you wouldn't start."

Then he proceeded to show me that I had not been inhaling! My "experience" with cigarettes was based on movie star glamour shots. I stopped pretending "sophistication" and am grateful to him for that advice. I hope that at some point you will be grateful to this book for helping you find the motivation you need to lose excess weight and keep it off.

While it is obvious how alcohol and drug addictions affect our loved ones, it has often been thought that obesity affects only the person who is overweight. Nothing, however, could be further from the truth. Speaking from experience, men and women who are overweight have a tremendous influence on their families.

My mother was a sergeant in the Women's Army Corps when she got pregnant with me. At that time a pregnant woman got an honorable discharge. The pregnancy was, of course, not planned and she was not happy about it. As I grew up she frequently reminded me of that fact.

Although I now know my mother loved me very much, that was not evident to me while growing up. There were no outward displays of affection. Her way of showing love was through food and entertainment.

Mother loved going to the theater, but the best we could do on her teacher's salary was stars of the silver screen movies. I think I saw The Sound of Music at least six times. When she found a movie that quickly became a favorite, she bought tickets for all of her friends (and mine) and we went numerous times.

She loved expensive restaurants, too. At the beginning of each month, after payday, we went to the nicest restaurants in San Antonio, Texas. (Later she said of me that I had "champagne tastes on a beer budget." I wonder why!) At the end of the month, when money was running out, she would cook a pot of stew and a pot of beans.

Thus, my idea of a "perfect" family was a wife/mother who was home when the children got home from school and a husband home from work with the smell of cookies or a pie in the oven waiting for them. I became that loving woman.

Friends who have known me through thick and thin would tell you that I was a gourmet cook and a perfect hostess. I willingly tried any recipe and the richer in fat and sugar the better. I remember making rolls of refrigerator cookie dough before you could buy it prepackaged and popping tray after tray of cookie dough into the oven for "hot-out-of-the-oven-melt-in-your-mouth" cookies for entertaining.

It was nothing unusual for me to buy a full longhorn of sharp cheddar cheese (6-pounds) and have it as a centerpiece with crackers or hot apple pie. When my husband went fishing (frequently), we would invite everyone over for a big fish fry. At other times it would be venison steaks or slow-smoked barbecue ribs.

Although I learned to cook by trial and error, and later country cooking with my mother-in-law, the meals I cooked were far from being nourishing or balanced. And, too often, when my daughter or son needed to talk, I put comfort food in front of them.

The result? Two children who learned to stuff their emotions with food and two overweight parents who had no skills in problem solving, communicating their emotions to each other, or knowing how to be there for each other or their children.

How much of my rollercoaster affair with weight can be attributed to control issues? A good deal of it. I felt I had no control over my own destiny both with my mother and my two husbands. The one thing that I could control was what I ate and I consistently made choices that, in hindsight, were self-destructive.

At the time, however, I could not see that I had any choices. This is easily explained by any one of several sociological and psychological models. Ones that I am most familiar with are Maslow's Hierarchy of Human Needs (psychology) and Spiral Dynamics (sociology).

In either model, a person or society that moves higher up the pyramid or spiral can look back at their past behaviors and easily see different choices they could have made, but didn't. Better choices? Possibly, but not necessarily. Just different choices.

While we're in the midst of our dramas, it is almost impossible for us to see healthier options. This is how a psychologist can help you. She or he can see solutions from an educated perspective and make a difference in your life if you follow their advice.

I escaped my mother's lifestyle by getting married and was a reasonably slender bride. I could just as easily have escaped by pursuing my business-related dreams. Instead, I plunged headlong into a marriage that was more or less happy for 3-4 years; then, disillusionment set in as I realized more and more that I would never be allowed to live my own dreams.

Sharon Kay, M.A., L.U.T.

Could I verbalize that realization? No. I couldn't even admit to being unhappy and sexually frustrated. That would have meant admitting failure.

Same thing, different scenario, with my second marriage. Yes, on the surface they looked different, but the realities of feeling that I had no control were the same.

Albert Einstein said that the definition of insanity is "doing the same thing over and over again and expecting different results." By that definition, I was insane the first 55+ years of my life!

With Unity I had an awakening. I learned what it meant to take control of my own life and be responsible for my own actions—past, present and future.

My son recently had gastric bypass surgery after reaching nearly 400-pounds. He is diabetic, was on four insulin shots a day and a walking pharmaceutical of prescription medicines. He has lost over 100-pounds as of this writing. Within two weeks he was off insulin and is now off all but one medication.

I felt a need to apologize to him before the surgery. Yes, he is an adult. And, yes, adults have to grow up at some point. Still, I felt that I had planted the seed of obesity throughout his childhood and I verbally tried to make amends. His reply, "I love you, Mom." Very few parents deliberately set out to ruin their children's lives and he knows that I love him.

I do not advocate surgical methods for weight loss, but my son is a walking example of the benefits that some people achieve from surgery. His wife, too, had weight reduction surgery and lost over 175-pounds. As a team I believe they will make it long-term.

My personal goal has always been, and still is, to retrain my mind and body. My son's environment and mindset were not conducive to doing so. Mine are and I believe most of you have that ability, too. I have come a long way, but there is room for improvement.

Last year a friend sent me a copy of a small booklet called *Happy Money* written in 2012 by Laina Buenostar. An exercise in learning how to manifest money is to write a letter to "Dear Spirit of Money and Abundance" apologizing for all of the negative thoughts and emotions I have had in that regard. I did ... and immediately began to notice results.

Then I wrote a letter to "Dear Men of the World" and, finally, one to "Dear Spirit of Food":

> *Dear Spirit of Food,*
>
> *I have had a negative image of you all my life. Rather than nourishment for my body I have used you as a narcotic to dull the pain of other issues.*
>
> *Finally I understand that you are good = God when used in moderation and making wise choices. I want to develop a positive relationship with you and I believe I am ready.*
>
> *I love and bless you.*
>
> *Sharon*

I invite you to write your own letter and free yourself from any negative emotions surrounding food.

NOTE: Two days after Thanksgiving 2015 my son sent me a text message apologizing for not calling on Thanksgiving day. He said that he had been sick—and that when he is sick now he is very, very sick. You see, after gastric bypass surgery you have no immune system to fight off germs and infections that our bodies usually handle routinely.

I know that his doctor explained every possible side effect to him while the decision-making process was going on. But can we totally understand the negative aspects of a procedure until after it is too late to change our minds?

Was the surgery worth it? I'm sure he will say it was, but I can't help but believe there was an easier way. My method of weight loss might seem as bad to him as withdrawal from a narcotic considering the large quantities of food he used to consume. But would moving past withdrawal symptoms be any worse than what he has gone through?

Only time will tell.

Sharon Kay, M.A., L.U.T.

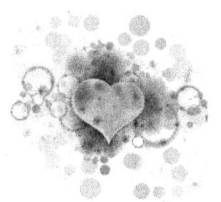

9: Compulsive Behaviors—
Weighing and Measuring

I have been taught, and I believe it is necessary, at least in the beginning, to weigh and measure everything that we are going to put in our mouths when at home. When I am at a restaurant I order items on the menu that have the calorie count listed and, if possible, I choose them on the Internet before going to the restaurant.

Last night, however, I recognized weighing and measuring as having being one of my compulsive addictions. I was the leader for a communion service at my church on Good Friday. That involved preparing the table with bread and wine (we use grape juice) and leading the congregation in the service.

It brought back memories of my early days in Weight Watchers when, while participating in a communion service, I would compulsively make allowances for the calories in the bread and grape juice and make sure I wrote them in my diary.

This time, after the service was over and there was lots of bread and juice left, we took it into the kitchen and had communal sharing. I picked up two of the tiny (probably one-half ounce) glasses of grape juice, one in each hand, and laughingly called myself a two-fisted drinker. I didn't eat any bread, because even pumpernickel is wheat-based.

Learning that I can stay on my program within reason, without counting every single calorie, frees me from the compulsive fear of losing control. The calories in the small amount of communion bread and grape juice (even wine if you are not in Alcoholics Anonymous) served during a service is not going to show up on the scale when you next weigh in.

Weighing and measuring is, however, a good habit to develop. And, interestingly, one of the main reasons to do so is to be sure that you are getting enough to eat. When a person is serious about losing weight, they often overestimate the number of calories or points they are consuming. Eating less than you need is not good for your health and you won't lose weight any faster.

After you have been weighing your servings of protein and vegetables that should be limited you will find that you can judge quantities pretty accurately without weighing. Doing so occasionally when you get to that point is, however, a good habit to cultivate. Is that an 8-ounce steak or a 3-ounce steak (about the size of a deck of cards)?

One form of weighing that should be limited is weighing yourself on bathroom scale every day—or sometimes many times a day. Both male and female bodies weight fluctuates and that fluctuation depends on many variables. What we eat and when we eat it, fluid retention, how much we have walked or not walked, medications we are talking and probably factors that I have not even considered because they were not pertinent to my body.

I have been taught to weigh once a week and, as much as possible at the same time of day. My preference is when I get up on Saturday morning before I get dressed, because that is when I am the lightest.

It does not matter, though, when you weigh as long as do it at the same time and in basically the same state of dress, or undress, every week.

NOTE: The good thing about Internet search engines is that you can find anything you need to find. The bad thing about Internet search engines is that you can find anything you need to find! When I did a search for "How often should I weigh while dieting?" I found numerous conflicting advice.

The bottom line: Once a week works best for me. Otherwise, I tend to see a good weight loss one day and tell myself that it gives me permission to eat anything I want to eat the next day. Not good!

Sharon Kay, M.A., L.U.T.

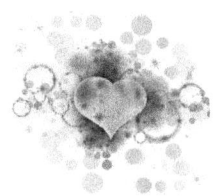

10: Compulsive Behaviors - Worry

In October 2013 my car caught on fire. I had been to church, picked up a church member to ride with me, and we noticed a funny sound all the way there and back. It sounded like it was coming from the area of the air conditioner and I assumed there was a problem with the motor.

As I dropped my friend off at her place I told her I would get it checked out the following week. I got to my home, pulled into my carport, turned off the engine, and black smoke poured out of the heating and cooling vent. Still I didn't worry, figuring I would go to my mechanic the next day after work.

The next morning I got up to go to work, started my car, and quickly realized that I had no power steering. Fortunately, I lived close enough to walk.

I spent about 30 minutes worrying.

In the past I might have gone into a compulsive pity party. Thoughts about how much I had in my emergency fund, how I wasn't really in a position to borrow money, etc., would have kept me awake.

Instead, I stopped and asked myself, "What would Jesus do?" The first thought I had was, "Well, he sure wouldn't spend any time worrying about it!" I stopped worrying and started doing what I do best—talking. I didn't ask anyone for anything, just talked about what had happened to the car.

Offers for help started pouring in. One man asked if I had AAA coverage. I didn't, but my insurance company includes roadside assistance and towed me to my mechanic's shop free of charge. A woman offered a loaner car if I needed it. I ended up not having to take her up on the offer. Another person offered money if I needed it. I had enough money in my emergency fund to cover the repair.

I was supposed to drive about 300 miles to meet a friend from Texas who was visiting her sister in Kansas on Thursday. I was back on the road and made the trip on schedule.

Imagine how much worse it could have been—especially considering that temperatures that week were down to -11° at times. What if I had been stranded on the side of the road in subzero temperatures? But I wasn't. I know beyond a shadow of a doubt that I am always divinely protected and that my role in that situation was to remain calm and allow the universe to roll out the red carpet for me. I did ... and it did. Thank you, God!

The old Sharon would probably have gained 10-pounds by eating every comfort food she could get her hands on to numb the pain of obsessive worry.

In my work I have heard prayers for every possible situation which invokes worry known to humankind. Among others I recall:

Germs	Children
ISIS	Global warming
Finances/Stock Market	Government/Politics
Genes/Heredity	

In Eckhart Tolle's book *The Power of Now* you are asked to:

"Focus your attention on the Now and tell me what problem you have at this moment."

He goes on to say that:

"...it is impossible to have a problem when your attention is fully in the Now."

While reading the book I realized that any worries I had came from something that had happened in the past that I could not change or something that could or would happen in the future that I had no control over. I made a conscious choice to no longer worry about anything that I can do nothing to prevent

Does that mean that I am like an ostrich with its head in the sand, apparently oblivious to what's going on around it? Actually, yes. You see, that ostrich is not oblivious. By keeping its ear to the ground it is very alert to any danger that may present itself.

While it may seem that I talk a lot, I actually listen more. By listening we learn and we keep our attention focused on the pulse of any situation that we may find ourselves in. Because of that, we are much more apt to act rationally and be able to make a real difference in an immediate crisis.

Sharon Kay, M.A., L.U.T.

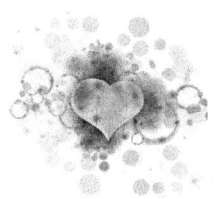

11: Compulsive Behaviors— Stress

At times of stress it is critical for me to be super organized in regard to what I plan to eat. What I have to remember at times like this is that psychologists recognize that stress comes in many different forms—positive as well as negative. This was well-documented by the Holmes and Rahe Stress Scale (1967) and numerous subsequent empirical studies. (See chart on page 210.)

Recently I had two career paths presented to me as options. Both appeared positive and both were of interest. I had not set out to look for a new job. These came to me which is always a good sign. Two friends, at different times, said, "Sharon, have you heard that the position of _____ is open?" (No.) "Well, you were the first person I thought about when I learned that it needed to be filled."

At the same time I found myself having oral surgery and unable to stay on my normal diet when the dentist ordered soft foods. Do you think I could stick to things like soups and applesauce? Of course not. It was a good excuse for homemade lemon meringue pie from a family-style restaurant—comfort food!

I found myself focusing on possibilities rather than planning meals. No, I didn't do any serious damage to my weight loss, but I felt out of balance and definitely broke my OA abstinence.

So what do you do when that happens? Get right back on the horse (or bicycle or ...) and continue to make positive progress. Learn from the experience. What did I learn this time? I learned how important having meals preplanned and sticking to that plan is to my success.

An experience I had over subsequent weeks showed me how very important structure is for me, too, in order to be able to maintain my weight loss schedule.

I joined a weight loss support group at work that meets 5-6 p.m. every Wednesday. That would be convenient since I usually eat dinner around 6 p.m. However, I have another group that meets 6-8 p.m. which has been an important part of my life for three years and I'm not willing to give it up.

Since I get off work at 3:30 p.m., I would either have to eat my evening meal around 4:30 p.m. (and that would be pushing it) or after 8 p.m. at night. Neither is an acceptable time for me to be able to go through the evening and not be hungry.

I realized that the extra meeting was throwing my schedule off not just for the one evening, but into the next day as well, and this was very stressful for me. Since it is extremely critical to me, on many levels, to maintain the pace of weight loss that I have set for myself as a demonstration, I notified the leader that I would no longer be a part of that weight loss group. I have my OA meeting on Saturday morning and that is sufficient to keep me focused.

NOTE: When we set our priorities and stick to them, divine grace often goes to work. When I spoke with the leader of the group, she said that Tuesday nights would work better for her. We talked to other group members and they were agreeable. So I get to have the best of both situations.

Even as I wrote the above section on the importance of structure in losing weight, I took a break from that structure. Go easy on yourself! There are times when our bodies just need a chance to take a break and catch up.

With all of the things that were going on in my life that you've just read about, I needed a sabbatical from weighing and measuring and watching every bite that went in my mouth.

Does that mean that I aimlessly ate any and everything that I wanted or everything that was presented to me at restaurants and parties? No. Actually, OA's plan that I adhere to says that I eat three reasonable meals a day, plus snacks of fruit. It does not say that I have to weigh and measure everything.

I followed the plan pretty well except during the healing from surgery, at which time I gained five pounds. However, I was able to release those added pounds in the two weeks following surgery in spite of not being structured. Normal people stop eating before they get uncomfortably full. By my definition, I was "normal" during this period.

You and I can do it!

After reading this section I know that I have the following issues to work on

_____

_____

_____

_____

_____

_____

_____

_____

_____

_____

_____

_____

_____

_____

_____

_____

_____

_____

_____

_____

_____

_____

Sharon Kay, M.A., L.U.T.

PART THREE

What Are

Your

Emotional Issues?

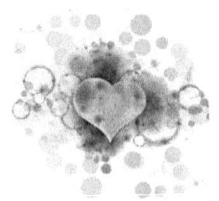

12: To Cut or Not to Cut

If you've ever weighed as much as I weighed at my maximum, you know that when you lose weight there is going to be excess skin. I have thought compulsively about what I would do when I was at my perfect weight. But making a decision is much more complicated than just getting over fear of major surgery.

Because I would like to be in a loving, committed heterosexual relationship at some point in the future, I have often wondered whether a man would prefer to have a woman with excess skin that is actually pretty or a woman with scars from having had the skin removed.

A coworker who had gastric bypass surgery also had cosmetic surgery to remove her excess skin. She showed me her scar which was barely noticeable; however, I will have a lot more excess skin.

Intellectually I know that this is very individual with different men and that I have to make my own decision based on what is best for me. I tell myself that I should be very happy with the fact that I look quite good in clothes. That, however, does not make it any easier for me to look at myself naked in the mirror!

Girlfriends tell me that most men couldn't care less about a woman's size as long as she has the right equipment and willingness to use it. That causes more emotional issues for me, because that means there is some other reason that I'm not in a relationship as I write this book. It is so easy to blame any issue on being overweight.

The decision on whether to have excess skin removed is not, however, limited to cosmetic concerns. Overlapping tissue can cause minor to serious health challenges. Heat and body oils combine to chafe epidermal layers and cause burn-like areas.

Unfortunately, this is an area that does not have many nerves so it really doesn't hurt. A person may not realize that serious damage has been done until after the fact and, therefore, the skin takes longer to heal.

According to www.naturalremedies.org/chafing, **"Those who are most obviously at risk for chafing are the highly physically active and the overweight, two groups who would normally have not much in common. In the case of athletes, any kind of poor fit in uniform can cause the skin to rub against the fabric of the uniform and cause chafing. As mentioned before, introducing moisture to the equation only intensifies chafing and makes it worse. Athletes tend to work out quite a bit and sweat profusely while doing so.**

"In overweight and obese people, skin often rubs against other skin in situations where people of average weight would not have to worry about this. The most common example of this is the fact that overweight people have much more thigh-on-thigh contact [and stomach skin overlap] and thus rubbing and friction than does an average person. **"Overweight people tend to become hot more quickly than smaller people and thus they sweat more easily. Athletes expect that they will produce large quantities of sweat and do so often, but it is impossible to predict when an overweight person might unexpectedly sweat and create an uncomfortable rubbing that can only be alleviated by changing clothes. If this happens while the overweight person is busy with work, school, or any number of other things that could prevent him/her from changing clothes, s/he could be stuck with sweaty areas that are primed to cause some painful chafing throughout the day."**

While cosmetic surgery to remove facial wrinkles or tummy looseness after a woman has children, removing excess tissue may not be as much cosmetic for the formerly obese individual as it is to improve ones health and well-being.

Unfortunately, many insurance companies still consider excess tissue removal to be cosmetic. If yours does what options do you have other than spending enough out-of-pocket money to build a small home? Major surgery like we're considering here is not cheap.

At one time I looked into donating excess skin to an organization like Shriners Hospital burn centers which seemed like a win-win situation. I understand that in the past they would actually pay for the surgery in return for the skin. However, it seems that scientific advances have made artificial substitutes much less expensive and more practical and easily available as they no longer buy human tissue.

Having had extensive medical work done in India, going to a country with which I am familiar would be my choice. Other countries offer what are now being called Medical Vacations, but I will discuss the country, and its people, with whom I have experience.

Surgery in India

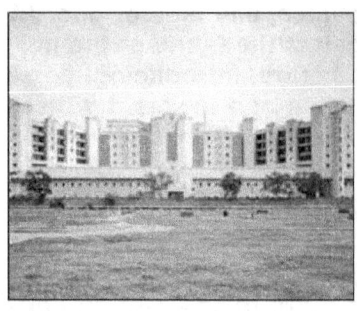

Indraprastha Hospital, shown in photograph at left, is an internationally accredited hospital in New Delhi, India, where I spent one night recovering from two surgical procedures.

It began in 2003 when I needed extensive dental restorations, including three bridges. Our company had people in India who did a large part of our computer work and I was very comfortable with the idea of them making arrangements for me.

Dental work that would have cost $15,000 in the United States cost $1,500 in India. Even with airfare, luxury 5-star hotel accommodations, shopping sprees, tours to iconic Indian sites such as the Taj Mahal and giving my hosts a bonus for devoting time to me, the restoration cost less than half what it would have cost in the U.S. An added bonus … my dentist back home was very pleased with the results.

Two years later my husband and I traveled to India and had executive health assessments done. Similar assessments at Baylor College of Medicine cost thousands of dollars. These consisted of two days of the most extensive battery of lab tests imaginable, including examinations and consultations appropriate to our ages and genders, for $250 per person. Included in the fee were three consultations with specialists, and more could be added, if necessary, for minimal cost.

I knew before I went that I needed a cystoscopy to explore my bladder. During testing a 4.2 cm gallstone was found. After discussing my options with two very professional, English-speaking doctors, they agreed that they could work together and do both surgical procedures at the same time since a cystoscopy requires general anesthesia. My urologist came in and operated on one end; then the second doctor came in and did minimally invasive laparoscopic gallbladder removal. I spent one night in an Indian hospital getting acquainted with a delightful roommate and her helpful family who also enjoyed getting to know an American woman.

Many people would cringe at the idea of having surgery in a "Third World" country, but my experience was very positive. Because medical staff in India recognize contagious diseases as part of their culture, sanitation practices are much more complex and adhered to than those I have witnessed, or friends and family have experienced, in hospitals in the U.S.

　　　　　　　　　　　　Sharon Kay, M.A., L.U.T.

Would I have excess skin removed in India? Yes, without having to think twice about it. I would happily spend my recovery time in an ashram with an English-speaking nurse to help me with my needs. The cost for a nurse would be minimal, and her help would alleviate any concerns I might have about my ability to communicate my needs.

I have good insurance now, however, and Medicare for hospitalizations. So, if they consider skin removal necessary surgery rather than cosmetic surgery, it might be more economical to have it done in the U.S.

Yes, there are other countries such as Mexico that offer inexpensive surgical procedures. The positive experiences I had in India, including the loving Indian people, give me plenty of reasons, however, to return to India and to them.

When considering cosmetic surgery, other questions you might ask yourself include:

Is beauty really in the eye of the beholder?

Is the cost of cosmetic surgery worth it to me?

A person considering surgery in India does need to give careful consideration to the facts that: 1) U.S. insurance policies, including Medicare, will not cover medical procedures done in foreign countries; and 2) doctors in India cannot be sued for malpractice.

The latter made me feel that my doctors had my best interests at heart, and were free to do their best for me, since they did not have to get permission from an insurance company and did not have to worry about being sued if something went wrong. Any surgery, anywhere carries with it an amount of risk.

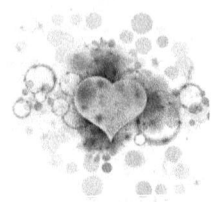

13: Fear of Success

The emotion of fear can masquerade in multiple ways, often leaving us feeling powerless or helpless. Neither is the truth. Perhaps the most insidious of those ways is fear of success.

As I was about halfway through writing this book, I found myself binge eating, gaining weight, and of course questioning the process.

I was getting rave reviews, not just about the book, but about other things that I was manifesting in my life and for other people. I had been recommended for two different jobs—neither of which manifested, leaving me with a feeling of disappointment, but neither of them were reflective of anything about me or my personality. One job was withdrawn from the marketplace. The other was postponed indefinitely.

I tried to find ways that I could stay in my current position, with decent benefits and salary, and still be able to promote this book and do other projects that I felt called to do. I learned that if I cut back to less than a 40 hour week I would not be entitled to benefits, though I could continue to work fewer hours.

A few weeks later, while getting ready for bed, my body ached … my mouth hurt from oral surgery previously mentioned—and I realized that I appear terrified!

It would have been so much easier to run and hide behind my comfort zone of fat. I talked with a photographer who was going to do glamour shots of me for the cover of this book—the first time in my life that I've ever done a photo shoot like this.

Silent Unity, where I can spend eight hours a day, five days a week, praying with callers, is safe. Implementing the plans I have for this book, for talks, workshops and extensive travel is more than a little intimidating.

It seems that I may be holding on tight to a fear of success. Yet I know it is time to release that fear. It is time to move out from behind the wall of insecurities I have built around myself—and being overweight is one way in which they manifested.

Sharon Kay, M.A., L.U.T.

Barbara Stanny, in her book *Secrets of Six-Figure Women* (2002), though referring to making financial changes in our lives, cautions **"Be forewarned. Anytime you do something new that runs counter to your prior conditioning, your habitual brain immediately responds: 'Watch out, this doesn't feel right! Stop immediately'."**

Sound familiar? Yes, it is just as pertinent to weight loss.

I believe the message I have been given is a message the world needs to hear. A message that you need to hear. Perhaps, I still need to hear it myself. I am beautiful. I am powerful. I am capable. I am successful. I am a winner!

(**NOTE:** I AM is humankind's spiritual name. It is a powerful statement of Truth and these two words should never be followed by anything negative because they give power to anything we claim. Thus, when we say, "I am fat," "I am stupid," "I am ...," we are claiming those things as true. I don't personally know most of you who are reading this book, but, without even seeing you, I know that the negative things you say about yourself are not your truth.)

- - - - -

Several months after writing the above section, my Power Posse group, based on Pam Grout's book, *E³* (pronounced E-cubed) (2014), did an exercise. Each of us had a few minutes during which we talked positively, affirming our dreams and aspirations.

When we were complete, other members of the group added their affirmations and visions to ours. It created a powerful energy that stayed with me and resulted in a decision to retreat into my apartment the following weekend for complete seclusion and silence.

I chose to continue using electronics which are an extension of my personality, but spent most of my time working on this book without the distractions of getting in the car and running errands, going to eat with friends, etc. An incredible amount of work was accomplished in a short period of time.

During this process the photographer for the cover of this book, Dawn Boomsa, reminded me of the "acting as if" principle promoted by Jack Canfield in his book, *The Success Principles! (2004).*

She suggested that I might affirm, "Ya'll, [she brought my Texas twang into this ☺] I can't believe I'm saying this, finally, but my book sold its *millionth* copy yesterday!!! I'm getting hundreds of emails from enthusiastic readers thanking me! I'm so excited I wanted to tell ya'll because next week I start my book tour next month!"

Dawn went on to remind me of a quote by my favorite author (a fact she did not know), Richard Bach, who said in *Jonathan Livingston Seagull*, "To fly as fast as thought, to be anywhere there is, you must first begin by knowing that you have already arrived."

Yes! I have arrived.

The following week our group did a "Come as if you have already arrived" exercise. I dressed in a tan gauze pantsuit, with red blouse and red high heels. Upon arriving I asked the hostess (prearranged) to set up a book signing table.

I had a mock-up of this book in hand and matching bookmarks with contact information on the reverse side. I "autographed" books and talked about how delighted I was at the large turnout, answered questions and, in general, had a wonderful evening—AND I announced that the millionth copy had sold that evening with the lucky winner receiving a free Loving to Lose retreat week (see advertisement at end of book) for themself or a friend.

Of course I helped others in the group imagine their successes, and everyone thoroughly enjoyed our visioning party. Try it ... you'll like it!

- - - - -

Perhaps I hadn't arrived quite as quickly as I thought.

The first week of 2016 I experienced pain on the right side of my body. I talked with my chiropractor about it, he did some testing, and said that it was a strain as if I had reached over my head for something and stretched too hard.

I didn't remember doing anything like that, and it actually didn't hurt most of the time. I could walk, I could lie down and sleep, I could sit at my desk at work and experience no pain. There was just a twinge of pain at times when I would do something that reminded me of the pain.

I began to analyze it metaphysically and realized that I have been stretching a lot—in writing this book and preparing to go on the road with it.

Metaphysically, the left side of the body is masculine; the right side is feminine. So it was my feminine side that was experiencing discomfort.

I quickly realized that it was as though I had two small children in my body who were arguing. (I am a Gemini and my twins sign can easily debate itself!). The little boy was excited and ready to get on the road and experience new adventures. On the other hand, the little girl was holding back—fear of the unknown, fear of success/failure.

Sharon Kay, M.A., L.U.T.

If had been simply a matter of changing jobs within the same geographical location there would have been no problem. As it was, I was considering (no, planning) a move into a career that would keep me on the road many weeks out of the year. I had to admit that, especially financially, with no guaranteed income it was scary even to my adult mind.

So I set my twin inner children down and talked with them assuring them that we could have the best of both worlds. We could go out and have fun and work with people and enjoy every minute of what we were doing. But we didn't have to do it all at once overnight. We could ease into it gradually, at a pace that was comfortable for both my inner girl child—and for me.

No surprise—the pain quickly disappeared.

Most of the time all that is necessary to release fear from an area of our lives is to: 1) recognize that it exists; and 2) face it head-on. Dream therapists tell us that if something frightens us during a dream that reaching out and grabbing hold of it will turn it into something that is not frightening. Same principle.

Note, however, that as long as these are any vestiges of fear that remain they will keep surfacing in different ways until they get our attention—such as mine did this time with physical pain—and the fear surfaced many times during the writing of this book. Each time I had to deal with it, recognizing that, as Franklin D. Roosevelt said in his inaugural address, "The only thing we have to fear is fear itself."

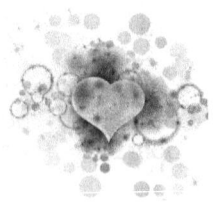

14: Looking for Love
for All the Wrong Reasons

While my first marriage probably began with a man being interested in my underage body, my second marriage was definitely about my brains. He had had a brain aneurysm and gone through a devastating divorce (which, in hindsight, was more devastating for her than it was for him) and I was quite literally his salvation from financial ruin. In hindsight, I thought he was my financial security.

We met in a professional organization and he was trying to figure out how he was going to move forward. What I didn't know at the time was that he was living by selling off assets while paying his former wife $2,000 per month to buy out her half of their assets.

I came along, with a job that would pay the wife, exceptional computer skills, a head for finances and, as it turned out, excellent sales abilities. Within a year I had resigned from my primary job, given up teaching college psychology classes, and soon gave up writing for a major newspaper which I loved in order to work full-time building what I perceived as our business. At the time of our divorce, I learned that he never did consider it *our* business, but rather *his* business—and apparently even my attorney agreed with him!

As I write these words, I am laughing. The fact that he had no morals, with either customers or with me, made my break from him easy. I never looked back and now recognize how necessary it was to my growth as a self-sufficient individual.

If my husband had done what he had promised, I would have given him credit (and probably half the royalties from my books). Instead, I learned to stand on my own two feet and now give myself and the God of my understanding the credit.

How is this pertinent to my weight loss? When I met this man I weighed nearly 300-pounds. The photograph you see of me on page 95 was taken on our honeymoon.

Sharon Kay, M.A., L.U.T.

He was tall, slender, owned his own home and had invested heavily in seriously valuable cars. On the surface, he could have had any woman he wanted. I've already described above why he was interested in me, but why was I interested in him?

I could see many of the problem areas. My boss at a crisis center for abused women and children tried to convince me that he showed signs of being an abuser. But I wouldn't listen.

In retrospect, I overlooked the negatives that were in plan sight in favor of an appearance of security. I vividly remember myself saying, "As long as I am willing to follow in his footsteps, I will go places I have never dreamed of going." And I did.

Was it worth it? Yes. It was necessary, just as being morbidly obese was necessary, for me to become the woman I am today. Could I have chosen another path? Yes, and I would have learned the same lessons. Perhaps they would have been gentler, but not necessarily.

We come into this world with what I would call "soul directives" which are not predestination, but rather experiences and emotions that we need for our spiritual development.

Once we have that experience, or experience a specific emotion, we are free to move on to other experiences and emotions. Take with you what you need from the experience of being morbidly obese, leave the rest behind, and emerge a more compassionate person for having had the experience.

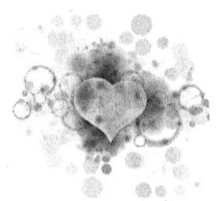

15: A Past-Life Made Me Do It

I have had some experience with past-life regressions and have come to believe that they are valid. If you would like to read my most dramatic experience, it is documented in a book I titled *Queen for an Hour: A Past Life Regression* which is available at www.amazon.com) However, two instances that are not in the book, which directly relate to my overeating in this lifetime, came to me through the help of psychic friends.

In one lifetime I was in Russia during a time of famine. In order to try to help our family, my husband had to go out on a ship. Unfortunately, something happened to him, I don't know what, and we never received any money from him. We had three children and we were starving. One of the children died.

In the second regression, I saw myself as a very verbal woman (imagine that) who opposed things in the church in colonial America. It got to a point where my husband and the minister of the church had me declared insane and committed to an asylum.

At the asylum another man and I fell in love. He was released and as soon as possible helped me escape. I could not go to my family so he and I went alone to a desolate area and lived in a cottage beside a lake. It was a good life and we grew old together.

When we got to an elderly age and realized we could no longer sustain our lifestyle, we talked about end-of-life choices. We elected to use the American Indian method of not eating any more. He died first and I followed soon thereafter.

If these lifetimes were realities, and I believe they were, is it any wonder that I came into this lifetime feeling starved and wanting to eat everything in sight? (Laughter)

A gaia (formerly GaiamTV) write-up about an interview with Jill Kuykendall, who is best known as a shaman who specializes in "soul retrieval" describes her work as:

"Have you ever suffered a serious accident, emotional

　　　　　　　　　　　　Sharon Kay, M.A., L.U.T.

trauma or loss from which feel you never fully recovered from the sense of having lost a part of yourself? Jill Kuykendall's life's work is helping people recover those lost parts with an ancient practice called soul retrieval.

Among indigenous people, it is generally understood that traumatic life experiences can fragment our inner, vital essence (soul) resulting in the loss or disassociation of soul parts that leave, carrying the burden of pain, shock, extreme emotion or memory of a trauma that are unbearable to the sufferer at the time. This fragmentation can occur in response to an obvious life trauma (post-traumatic stress syndrome experienced by military veterans is a classic example), or from a subtle troubling experience so personal to an individual that no one else would know that a trauma had occurred."

Starving to death would be a pretty traumatic experience!

The video is available at www.gaia.com/video/jill-kuykendall-soul-retrieval for a nominal membership fee which entitles you to watch anything Gaia has to offer.

A song, Shaman Woman, vividly takes you into Kuykendall's world. It was written by a dear friend, Gary Johnson, and is included on my Shape Shifting Meditation CD.

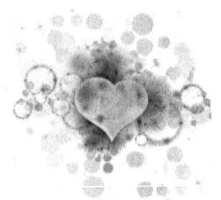

16: Embarrassing Moments?

"Aren't you embarrassed to be talking about being fat?"

Being overweight is a condition that many people throughout the world find themselves in. The alcoholic who is in recovery is praised for being able to admit that he or she has no control over alcohol and has turned their life over to a Higher Power.

And yet, being overweight is much harder to conceal than alcoholism. Why should I be embarrassed about having found an answer that can potentially benefit millions of people?

My embarrassing moments are in the past. I can recall many times when my weight embarrassed me. Two that come to mind are trying to ride a rollercoaster with my son when he was young. He was too young to ride by himself. When I got on with him, they tried to fasten the bar over my lap—and it was impossible. I was mortified and he was in tears about not getting to ride.

And of course there are always seatbelts on airplanes. It is bad enough that the seats are so small that a person who weighs more than 150-pounds is miserable flying economy class. On my honeymoon flight to England, I had to ask for an extender seat belt. I was mortified—but at least it didn't bring my husband to tears!

I am proud of myself now. I recognize that, in Overeaters Anonymous terminology, I am and always will be a compulsive overeater. That does not mean that I do not have the ability to live a normal life. Just as an alcoholic must turn away from alcohol in order to maintain sobriety, I have to say no to overeating, but that is not a death sentence. It is, rather, the path to a happy, healthy lifestyle.

Sharon Kay, M.A., L.U.T.

After reading this section I find that it really bothers me that _____

_____

_____

_____

_____

_____

_____

_____

_____

_____

_____

_____

_____

_____

_____

_____

_____

_____

_____

_____

_____

_____

PART FOUR

What Are

Your

Physical Issues?

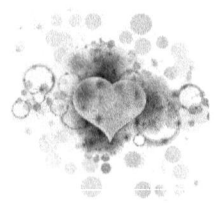

17: The Power of Imagination

Unity cofounder, Charles Fillmore, identified what he called "The Twelve Powers of Man" (www.unity.org/twelve-powers). Each power must be activated in order to be effective in our lives and each power later came to be associated with a month. I was born under the power of Imagination and anyone who knows me very well has no doubt that I was born with it fully active.

In the 1980s *Creative Visualization* by Shakti Gawain captured my imagination and changed my life. Two girlfriends and I joined forces and designed posters following Gawain's instructions for the purpose of creating our futures.

Today I use a different method of visualization, but it is simply a variation of Gawain's work and I still give her credit. The image on the opposite page is a sample page showing my desires for my spiritual life. I find it interesting that I, in my imagination (though perhaps not yours), am coming to look much like the woman on the staircase to heaven.

Recently I attended a film and discussion group which featured a GAIAM TV interview of Dr. Joe Dispenza on his latest book *You Are the Placebo: Making Your Mind Matter* (2015).

In an online summary of the book by Dawson Church, Ph.D., he says that, **"We're all inspired by such stories of spontaneous remission and 'miraculous' healing, yet what Joe shows us in this book is that we are all capable of experiencing such healing miracles. Renewal is built into the very fabric of our bodies, and degeneration and disease are the exception, not the norm."**

Church goes on to say that Dispenza gives his **"account of an accident that shattered six of the vertebrae of his spine. Suddenly, in extremis, he was confronted with the necessity of putting into practice what he believed in theory: that our bodies possess an innate intelligence that includes miraculous healing power. The discipline he brought to the process of visualizing his spinal column rebuilding itself is a story of inspiration and determination."**

Sharon Kay, M.A., L.U.T.

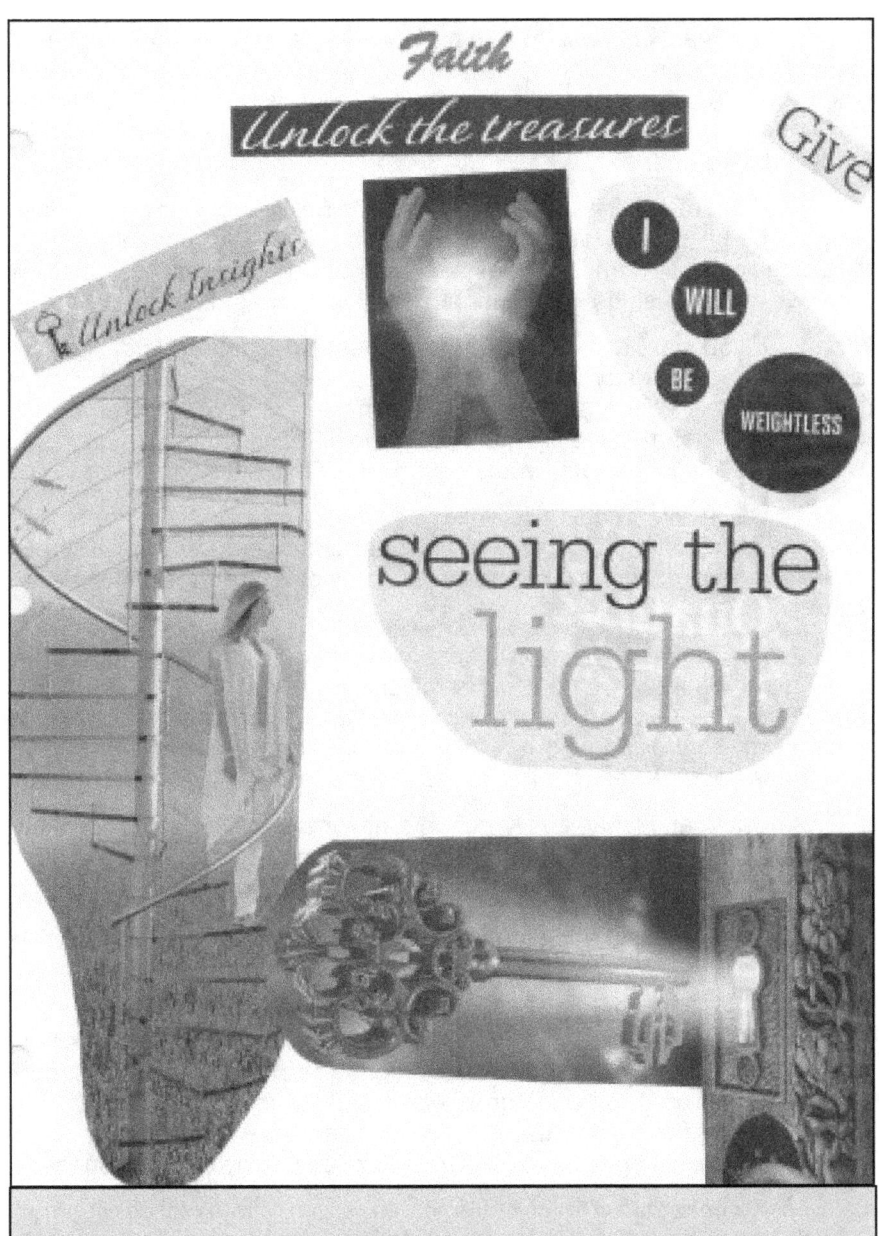

Page from my
Creative Visualization book

If a man who was told that he would never walk again can re-generate his spinal column, how much easier should it be for us to shed 75, 100, 200-pounds or more? I challenge you to allow your consciousness to rise to the point of believing it is possible and allow your body to be healed.

Dispenza talks about healing from illnesses, our physical challenges, by pretending as if (sounds like Jack Canfield, doesn't it) that challenge is just as important as any area of our lives that we want to improve—relationships, health, finances, career, weight loss, etc.

If you want to excel in any area, healing mind and body, acting as though you already have what you desire is a powerful tool. Unity has called this concept "fake it 'til you make it" for years. Rev. Paul Hasselbeck, dean of the Spiritual Education & Enrichment program at Unity World Headquarters, would change it to "faith it till you make it."

While this concept is valid, and one that can be understood perhaps better by individuals in traditional churches, the truth is that, when we are trying to manifest something, it often feels like we're faking it!

As I discuss with you steps I am taking to create a new Sharon—mind, body and career—it is difficult for me to understand that I am already the person I am striving to create. The person I see looking back at me in the morning is a persona that I have chosen to put on, and it has become very familiar to me. It feels real.

But I can just as easily put on a new persona. In fact, a teacher and mentor recently said to me, "It feels as though I am seeing the real Sharon for the first time."

It is true. I am chipping away the protective shell of insecurities that had become crystallized around me and am allowing the reality of who I am in my mind, heart and soul to be revealed.

Admittedly, as I write this section, the woman on the cover of this book is not yet "reality" to me. Though the photographs are not Photoshopped, a good photographer, telling me to "tuck your butt in," pull your stomach in, and using proper lighting can work miracles. It is me ... yet those images have not yet crystallized in my consciousness.

A concept that I am attracted to is the Many Worlds Theory. The hypothesis is that all potential exists at the same time. The 296 1/2 -pound Sharon exists at the same time as the 175-pound Sharon. My thoughts, words and actions decide which of the two women the world sees at any given time.

It is best explained in James Twyman's book *The Barn Dance*. Twyman writes the book as though it were fiction, but explains in the introduction that "... for me it is absolute truth."

In the book he visits an area where dimensions of existence intersect and steps into another of his own realities. In discussing their lives with his former wife who had been murdered three years earlier, she explains:

"There is no particular *look* or *way of looking* here. You are seeing me in the way I once was, but now none of that matters. You could see me as a child, or when I was forty-three. I'm not limited to any of that, just as you are not limited to the way you look right now." (pg. 92)

"... there are aspects of you that live one adventure and other aspects that do something completely different. That's because we live in a universe that's dynamic and unlimited. Nothing moves in straight predictable lines ...." (pg. 122)

When I look in my mirror at home I see a different woman than I see when I am surrounded by the energy of people who love, even like me. My "reality" which manifests in the world appears different than the woman who stares at me when I awaken each morning.

Twyman's wife says that, **"You can only be consciously aware of one, but you are experiencing both at the same time."** (pg. 183)

According to my interpretation of Twyman's book, what this means is that every Sharon Kay that could possibly exist actually does exist at the same time.

When you meet me for the first time, why do you see me as you do? There are many possible explanations. One I can comprehend is that I am focusing on this "me"; thus, that image manifests. Another is that you are seeing the "me" that you expect to see after having read my book.

Thank you for giving me the impetus and the energy—even before you meet me—to bring to light an image I love presenting to the world. It has nothing to do with cosmetics because the only makeup I wear is a touch of lipstick—occasionally. It has nothing to do with the way I style my hair or the clothes I wear.

It has everything to do with the energy exchange between us.

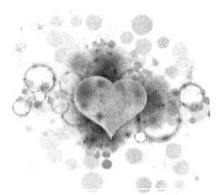

18: Importance of a Clear Vision

In using our imagination, it is important to examine all aspects of what we want—not just physical, but mental, emotional and spiritual as well. I wanted a slender man, who had done well in business, for my future husband. Using Gawain's techniques discussed in the previous chapter, I got exactly what I asked for.

The number one lesson I learned ... be careful what you ask for—you will get it! I did. Travel, my writings published, weight loss and the husband of my vision boarding.

I had a collage of photographs showing travel by plane, train, boat and car. I subsequently flew to India and Europe, rode the high speed rail in Europe, owned and drove a Porsche Boxster convertible, and test drove exotic collector cars such as a DeLorean Gullwing coupe (think "Back to the Future" movies) at a collector car meet and a Bentley T sedan on Silverstone Race Track in England.

Within nine months I attracted a man who looked exactly like the man in the picture, who was in the same profession. He was slender. He had done well in business (keywords "had done") and it had fallen apart due to a recession in his industry. On top of that, he almost died from a brain aneurysm. Louise Hay, author of numerous books including *You Can Heal Your Body*, cites brain tumors as resulting from "Incorrect computerized beliefs. Stubborn. Refusing to change old patterns." It fit him like a comfortable old glove!

During his illness he felt that his wife had deserted him and he filed for divorce. I met him a little over a year later. Of course I heard his side of the story and blamed her.

Interestingly, his best friend tried his best to talk me into a prenuptial agreement. I argued that he was the one who had all the assets—a prenuptial was simply saying that he didn't trust me. Too late, I realized that the man was trying to protect me from his friend!

I attracted exactly the husband I had put on paper and nothing more. I got a paper man, a man incapable of feeling empathy for anyone other than himself. Oh … he could feel emotion if he felt that he had been wronged. But if he wronged someone else, he believed it was their fault, not due to any action of his.

I found that I wanted and needed more. I needed intangibles that are not easily recorded on poster board or in a book. I needed someone who was capable of feeling emotions other than anger, someone who was loving and giving, someone who was secure in their own abilities and manhood. He had none of those qualities.

His beliefs included a sense of entitlement. He felt he had a right to walk all over someone if they didn't play the game his way.

While writing this book I got a call from an attorney representing a man who wanted to file a business lawsuit against my former husband. I found myself wanting to help them! I know how it feels for this man to cheat you. Even though I didn't have the information they were looking for, I could tell them how he operates.

What I have learned, though, is that it wasn't his fault. I was attracted to him, and imagined that I saw in him the qualities I was looking for in a man. In hindsight I recognize that I was creating an image that was not his reality. As of this moment, unless the attorney calls me again, I will not act on my ego's prodding. (They did. I answered their questions and the lawsuit was settled out of court without further involvement on my part.)

In order to attract, or be attracted to, the person we really desire in our heart, we must first be that person ourselves. Then and only then will we be able to recognize the person whom I have come to call my Twin Flame.

If you want a man in your life who is spiritual, creative, loving, giving, compassionate, interesting, fun to be around guess what qualities you need to develop in yourself? Similar interests, or a real interest in the other person's interests and abilities, are good, too. I was attracted recently to a man who loves the outdoors. My idea of being "outdoors" is enjoying a manicured garden through plate glass windows!

How does this work? They say that opposites attract, but do you want to be with someone who wants to sit home in front of the TV when you want to go hiking? Wouldn't you rather be with someone who enjoys hiking with you? Do you want to be with someone whose favorite meal is beer and hamburgers when you like steak and shrimp (or worse yet, you are vegetarian or vegan)?

Sure, you can make it work, but it is work. And you will do most of the work. The only person we can change, or have a right to try to change, is ourself.

How much better would it be to be clear on what we need and want in a relationship; and then make sure that we are already in that relationship—with ourselves? At that point, we will find ourselves going to places and events that someone like us would attend.

Voila! A magical encounter. Imagine that! Well, why not? You created the magic!

Attracting or manifesting, including weight loss, can be easy if we use our imagination to make a fun game of something most people consider torture. For example, think of something that you are looking forward to—perhaps a trip, a date, a graduation or retirement. Then close your eyes and visualize yourself in that setting and looking the way you want to look. See the way you will dress, the things you will do.

You are at your perfect weight. You move lightly, gracefully, with ease. You see someone you know and they come to hug you, complimenting you on how good you look. A tray of appetizers is offered—you wave it away, knowing that the conversation you are having is much more satisfying than any appetizer would taste.

Imagination can be stimulated through interactions with other people who are capable of seeing the Truth of who you are ... a beautiful child of the Universe. These people are usually not family and friends who are close enough to see all your shortcomings (also known as "warts").

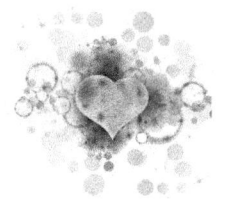

19:Find an Overeater's Anonymous (OA) Meeting

A good place to find support for your weight loss efforts amidst people who can help you visualize a new you is a weight loss support group. How members look, talk and live their lives are very important factors to consider Personally, I have a problem with someone trying to teach me how to lose weight who, obviously, has not done the work themself.

I am going to discuss Overeater's Anonymous (OA) here because there are no leaders and the group will not try to teach you how to lose weight. What attending meetings will do is give you mental and emotional support and, by working their 12 Steps, help you figure out why you are eating 3,000 calories a day when you only need 1,200. The cost is a love offering which truly means giving what you can afford based on the value the meeting brings to you.

There are thousands of OA meetings throughout the world, but if there isn't one near you, there will be one online (www.oa.org/membersgroups/find-a-meeting) where you can admit to being a compulsive overeater and chat with people who have similar challenges.

I know that if you only need to lose 15-pounds it may be difficult to admit to compulsive overeating, but if those extra pounds are bothering you, or affecting your health, there is a reason you are not losing them. It has been said that words are cheap, but sometimes they're painful to say. Admitting that you are a compulsive overeater is the price you pay to get the most out of this program.

A group like OA is especially critical if you are in a toxic home environment. For some of us it is just on holidays or at family reunions. You know, the times when Aunt Jane insists that you sample her homemade pecan pie. "One little piece (1/6 of the pie) won't hurt." At the same time you are bombarded by Aunt A's cake, Aunt B's potato salad, Uncle D's fried chicken, Uncle E's barbecue ... and on and on, ad nauseum.

Are you on the receiving end of this abuse at other times, too?

Does your husband insist that he can't live without chips and beer in the house. Or perhaps you have kids who demand Twinkies for their lunch boxes and sugar-coated cereals for breakfast—because all their friends do (doubtful).

If any of the above scenarios describe your environment, you desperately need to give yourself the gift of a support group. I recommend OA because it is basically free, but any group that provides loving, non-judgmental support is fine. It could be at church. It could be at your public library. You could start your own as Jean Nidetch, founder of Weight Watchers, did.

And the OA "plan" is quite simple. Find a healthy weight loss method that you think (or know, as I know that a basic Weight Watchers plan works for me) will work for you and stick to it. When you do ,you are considered to be "abstinent." When I first heard that word several years ago at an OA meeting in Texas (I went to only two meetings.), I thought, "Sure ... that's good advice for an alcoholic. But how do we abstain from food? We have to eat."

I was given a book entitled *Abstinence*, but I'm pretty sure that I couldn't get past that word and never read the book. This time I did. This time I learned that many people in OA choose a plan which requires them to eat three moderate meals a day. If they eat anything outside the plan it is considered breaking abstinence.

My plan is three moderate meals a day, for which I keep detailed records (and thus this book was born), plus a snack of fruit at each of my breaks during work hours. I found the fruit to be necessary for me because I eat breakfast at 6:30 a.m. and lunch usually isn't until 1:30 p.m. That's too long for our bodies to be without any new nutrition. Even if you are not diabetic, blood sugar levels affect how you feel and productivity on your job, whether you are a stay-at-home mom or an executive.

I pack a lunch box for work the night. As long as I don't raid the vending machine or have a bite of celebratory cake (nearly every day Is a celebration of some sort) that someone has brought in and eat only what I brought with me, I am abstinent.

This flexibility is necessary for me because my lunches and breaks are not set in stone. In fact, the week I wrote the above about lunch being at 1:30 p.m.. it was changed to 10:30 a.m.

Around 6 p.m. I eat my third planned meal either at home or at a restaurant with a friend. The rest of the time, other than simple shopping and preparation time, I think of things more important than food.

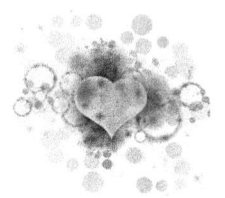

20: Keep a diary of Your Habits

As your support system develops, begin taking time to analyze your eating habits.

What do you eat, when and how much? (see sample diary pages on pages 74-76 and charts in Meals, Menus and More section.) Are you usually alone or with family or friends? If you work, is there a communal room where people bring doughnuts, cakes, cookies, etc., to share? Are there potluck meals? When you get home from work do you have a meal planned or do you turn the television on and start a "minute I hit the door to minute I go to bed" binge (with midnight raid on the refrigerator)?

One thing keeping records does is help you establish your baseline—where you are at this point in time. The first thing I discovered when I started being honest with myself was that I grabbed a bag of chips (or candy or canned cake frosting!) when I first got home at 3:30 p.m. (after eating lunch at 1:30) and nibbled at the computer, or while reading or watching a movie, without ever sitting down to a planned meal.

Thankfully I was also very active and had meetings several nights a week which prevented me from munching non-stop until bedtime every day of the week.

Once I started planning a meal that could easily be put on the table at 6 p.m., and ate it, I found that I wasn't hungry the rest of the evening. Midnight peanut butter out of the jar raids are a thing of the past.

It also helps identify your triggers, which may not be food related. Soon after affirming that 2015 was going to be "The Year of Sharon" I found myself at a "Meet the Author" gathering in a friend's home for an introduction to Pam Grout's book, E^3. I thoroughly enjoyed the evening.

Pam sat down and talked with me before I recognized her as the guest of honor and told me that whatever I desired in my heart was already accomplished. I just had to recognize the Truth of that statement. And I did.

In addition, people from work who like, admire and respect me (and it is mutual) were there and I visited amicably with them. So why, the minute the talk was over, did I make an excuse to leave (run), grabbing a handful of pot stickers to munch on as I drove home? We had a full meal so it certainly wasn't hunger.

I recognized that my insecurities come out like monsters in the night when I am surrounded by people with Ph.D. after their name or Rev. before their name. As individuals I can and do interact comfortably with any of them and, in fact, I have as much or more education than some of the ministers

It was the energy of ghosts from the past that attacked me.

I wasn't consciously aware of it at the time, but in hindsight I can hear my mother, my first husband, my second husband, and other people who were in positions of control who, for one reason or another, led me to believe that I could never live up to their image of me. Thus, I was actually living "down" to their image of me.

There were other people, though, through the years, who were able to see in me the truth of my being. I vividly remember my sociology professor in community college praising my writing. "I always wait until I have time to read one of your papers from cover-to-cover before I start," she said, "because once I start I don't want to put it down."

Why is it that the ghosts of negative remarks come out to haunt us instead of the spirits of praise and encouragement? That's kind of like why do we crave chocolate instead of broccoli!

Last night I had a dream. I got to church in time to do the sermon. That's DO the sermon, not attend the sermon! I was the minister.

When I walked in the door I noticed that one of my old ministers was in the audience. Suddenly I couldn't remember how to do anything. My computer equipment didn't work properly. The service was to start on the hour and when I looked at the clock it was 15 minutes after, etc.

So many times in my life I have self-sabotaged. I know what I'm capable of doing, I know I am competent, and yet those little gremlins get ahold of me and I feel like I'm still in grade school!

Whether or not you have a position which requires public speaking, or whether you have any desire to do so, you know what I'm talking about.

Sharon Kay, M.A., L.U.T.

It is the gremlins that come out when you are visiting your parents and suddenly you feel like you are five years old and can't do anything right. It is the voice of your former husband telling you that you are lazy. It is any negative words or emotions that you've experienced throughout your lifetime—and claimed as your own.

Stop!!! Negativity has no power over us unless we allow it to!

You are not your parents. You are not anyone from your past who did not have your best interests at heart. You are not anything negative. You are a beautiful, capable child of the universe.

We cannot change anyone else unless they want to be changed, and then they need to do the changing themselves without being nagged. We can, however, change anything about ourselves—physical, mental, emotional or spiritual—that is not empowering us.

Collective energy from my past had attacked me with "You are not good enough" ... "You don't belong" ... "Who do you think you are?"

Of course, none of it is true and none of the people present at the event would have thought it, much less said it. It is ghosts from my past—ghosts that I allowed to drive me to an all-week binge. Fortunately, I was able to confess the emotions at an OA meeting; then immediately get back on my plan. It appears that healing of this issue has occurred.

Who/what ghosts do you need to confront? It is an interesting psychological fact that when we confront things we fear, whether in our everyday world or in nightmare dreams, they turn into something harmless—even sweet, loving, friendly.

SAMPLE PAGES FROM MY DIARY—
EARLY DAYS ON PLAN

January 5, 2015

I am very proud of myself today. I ate lunch in the break room where someone had brought in all kinds of chips, dips and hummus. Before I finished everyone else had left the room. I did not get into any of the offerings. I had eaten a full meal ... but that would not have stopped me in the past. It felt better today *not* overeating.

I feel kind of weak this evening. I don't think it is surprising since I'm down from probably 3000-4000 calories per day to 1200. But it is not like I have any hard labor to do so will continue on my abstinence plan and eat a regular meal at 6:00.

Also, I'm feeling a bit constipated which, again, is not surprising. My body will adjust.

I realized later tonight that eating less had nothing to do with the way I was feeling. Last night I had so many ideas going through my mind that I couldn't sleep. The last time I looked at the clock it was 1:30 a.m. No wonder I was tired. Tonight I took ibuprofen and went to bed at 8:00 p.m.

January 6, 2015

A coworker said this morning that I was "glowing." I feel light and healthy and happy. I feel in control—and that in itself may be an issue. I grew up with a mother who had been a sergeant in the Army when she got pregnant with me and blamed me for ruining her life. She was very controlling, but overweight, and food was the only area in which I felt that I had control over.

Until recently I wasn't so much different. Two marriages were disasters as I look back.

Now, however, my life is under control enough that I find myself relaxing at home instead of always being "on stage."

January 7, 2015

I feel so good today. Walked 10 minutes on first break instead of eating fruit. Chiropractor yesterday changed me from monthly to every other month appointments. I don't experience pain. He has been working on spinal alignment. Now that I am standing up straight I look like I weigh less than I do.

I had cereal with 3 T. dairy-free creamer for breakfast. It was very satisfying. The cereal was wheat-based, but I am not locked into the compulsion of absolutely no wheat. I am not allergic, but find that I feel better when I limit wheat. Abdominal bloating goes away and I feel lighter.

January 8, 2015

In 1995/96 I lost 100 lbs. and ended up having to have hernia surgery which led to Interstitial Cystitis which took three years to diagnose and, after getting rid of ulcers in the bladder, greatly diminished my capacity. I think one of my problems with losing weight is concern about messing up my balance again.

Then, too, there is the idea of all the excess skin that will need to be removed (I think) after losing 75 lbs. or more now.

I am walking easier, however, when I take 10-minute walks during one of my 15-minute breaks.

January 10, 2015 - 248.8# (-4.4)

I lost 4.4 lbs. last week. I could wish it were more, but the important thing is that I did so without feeling deprived and my clothes and my rings fit as though there was a much larger loss. The latter, I think, is due to being relatively wheat-free.

January 11, 2015

Church had two services with presentation of my L.U.T. certificate *and* food afterward for both services. I socialized and didn't eat a bite. I had lunch and dinner prepared and ready for me at home. Feeling good about staying on my plan felt much better than a piece of cake would have tasted.

It was a wonderful day!

January 12, 2015

A friend brought a chocolate cake to work for her birthday. Chocolate is not my favorite. I had 1/2 a grapefruit and kept cake behind where I was sitting.

Tomorrow "snacks" are being brought to celebrate my graduation and another friend's. I am planning a small sweet to go with my lunch. (Ended up taking a mini scone home and having it with a rich cup of coffee for an evening dessert. Excellent and on plan.)

My clothes are fitting much better and I look forward to smaller sizes.

<u>January 17, 2015</u> - 246.8# (-5.4)

Lunch at IHOP would have been considered a disaster in the past because I did not plan ahead. I had a chorizo omelet and fruit dish. When I got home I looked up calories and points and they were more than I should have had the entire day.

However, it was one meal out of three. I did not beat myself up and did not use it as an excuse to eat whatever I wanted to eat the rest of the day (week?). I went ahead and had a normal (small) planned meal in the evening, knowing that I will probably still lose a pound or so in spite of the lunch being more calorie/point intensive than it needed to be.

I enjoyed every mouthful!

Sharon Kay, M.A., L.U.T.

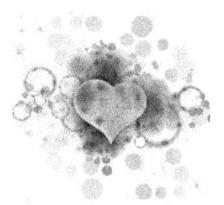

21: Know What You are Putting into Your Body

My mother, as previously mentioned, did as little cooking as possible. She taught school and both of us ate school lunches five days a week. At night we ate dinner out—luxurious restaurants at the beginning of a pay period and working our way down to the two meals she would cook as money ran out, a pot of beans and a pot of stew.

Oh yes, I almost forgot. She also cooked breakfast: a working farmer's breakfast of eggs fried in grease, bacon or sausage, and canned biscuits loaded with butter and jam!

I learned to cook pretty much in self-defense ... and all the wrong things. Cookies, pies, cakes all brought praise for my cooking from friends my mother's age and I basked in the compliments. Though mother didn't cook, she encouraged me by buying cookbooks for me and ingredients I needed to "experiment."

On my 18th birthday I married into a loving large family after having been an only child. I loved my in-laws, got lots of positive attention and learned to cook "country style." Typical meals were fried, creamed, salt and sugar laden. Until I join Weight Watchers, I thought the only way to cook fish was fried with sides of fried potatoes, fried okra, fried hush puppies and fried green tomatoes.

Today the word "fried" has pretty much been eliminated from my vocabulary, though I will stir-fry or brown vegetables in a minimal (1/2 teaspoon per serving) amount of coconut oil. The lighter and easier to prepare, the better it is for me ... and you. Heavy, dense is out. Light, high nutrition is in.

So ... and be honest, do you have any idea what you are fueling your body with? Or do you stop at McDonald's on the way to work for a breakfast sandwich and a latte, eat a fast-food lunch at your desk, and pick up a bucket of fried chicken with french fries or potato salad and coleslaw for your family's evening meal?

Check out the following sample menu that I used to eat.

ANALYSIS

McDonald's - http://nutrition.mcdonalds.com/getnutrition/
nutritionfacts.pdf

BREAKFAST: Bacon, Egg & Cheese Bagel with Egg Whites—

560 calories/12 points

McCafé Mocha (small)—340 calories—8 points

Panera Bread - https://www.panerabread.com/content/dam/
panerabread/documents/nutrition/Panera-Nutrition.pdf

LUNCH: Chilled Shrimp & Soba Noodle Salad (full)—

700 calories/18 points

(**NOTE:** Salads are good for you, right? Shrimp is low in calories, high in protein, and good for you, right? This salad has 39g protein (good), but it also has 87g carbohydrates (mostly from the noodles) and 22g fat!) Remember that a fat gram at 9 calories per gram means that 198 calories are from fat. At least Paneras lists calorie counts for all menu items, so you can choose to make a better choice.)

KFC - http://www.kfc.com/nutrition/

DINNER: Chicken Thigh (Extra Crispy), Potato Wedges, Coleslaw and

Biscuit—1010 calories/32 points

(NOTE: This meal is what I used to get at KFC, though I often had two chicken thighs, and the points value is what I should have TOTAL in a day's time. I also noted on the website that it does not list grams of fiber. We all know that our bodies need fiber for elimination, don't we? So why isn't fiber listed? Because most of their choices have very little fiber content.)

Sharon Kay, M.A., L.U.T.

At the end of this day I would have consumed 2050 calories and 58 points. That's not counting the doughnut(s) or birthday cake someone brought to the office that I "need" to carry me from breakfast to lunch. It doesn't count the numerous teaspoons of sugar in sodas and/or cups of coffee either.

When I met the man who would become my second husband, and we decided to live together, he handed me a list of simple foods. I thought he was telling me that it was all he would eat. Quickly, however, I learned that the list was all he expected: frozen pancakes, grits (southern), rice mixes, Cornish hens and other things I don't remember.

On our first grocery shopping trip together, I learned that we both loved liver and onions and I began to expand his list dramatically since, in some circles, I'm considered a gourmet cook.

As I said previously, I learned a lot during this marriage about my relationship with food by observing a "normal" (in the sense of dietary habits) person's relationship with food. Much of that has been carried forward to the present.

Today I know exactly what I'm putting into my body and why. I plan in advance, knowing that evening activities may require adjusting morning and afternoon intake.

I've also learned to forgive myself quickly and easily for any dietary indiscretion and immediately get back on track. Going on a weeklong binge following breaking abstinence is no longer an option. Well ... most of the time. On week 10 I started the week with two glasses of wine Saturday afternoon, nibbled my way through Sunday without counting calories or points, and on Monday my kitchen weighing scales went out. I immediately ordered a new battery, but that was a good excuse (NOT!!) to nosh my way through the entire week.

Yet I gained only one pound. This tells me that I made more good choices than I thought, because I no longer believe in "luck" on the scale (or in any other aspect of my life). I believe I am what I eat in regard to the appearance of excess pounds on my body. In the Meals, Menus and More section you will find sample pages from my daily calorie count/points count log.

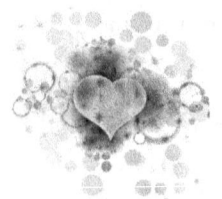

22: Variety—The Spice of Life

I get bored really easily! When I go to a smorgasbord, I want a little bit of everything (which turns out to be a heaping plate full—with seconds).

What I've had to learn is to: 1) avoid smorgasbords; and 2) buy and prepare small amounts of an assortment of foods to give me the variety I need without going over my nutritional limits.

So I will get, for example, a one-half pound portion of lean ham at the deli (remember that I am cooking for only one person) and pair four ounces with homemade (from a mix) scalloped potatoes and green beans for lunch or dinner. The next day the ham may be a sandwich with lettuce and tomato (and onion if I'm at home), chopped into a salad, or combined with different vegetable and starch options.

When you begin to think this way, it is possible to make many different meals out of a small quantity of protein, vegetables, and starches.

And don't, literally, forget the spices. One day a chicken thigh or breast can be Italian, the next day Mexican, the next day Indian. There are many dry rubs that have very few calories, and there are sauces so flavorful that you only need 1-2 tablespoons to flavor the meat.

If you feel that you don't have enough quantity when you first start eating for your health, add extra green vegetables and fruit which Weight Watchers counts as 0-point items. I limit those, too, but only because I have come to prefer feeling 80% full rather than feeling uncomfortably stuffed.

Sharon Kay, M.A., L.U.T.

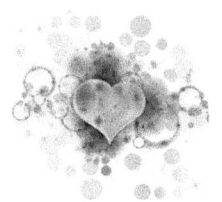

23: Drinking and Dieting

No, you don't have to give up your beer or wine ... but be aware that, on a 1200 calorie diet, a six-ounce glass of wine uses up one-tenth or more of your daily calorie allotment.

The author of an article on www.winefolly.com says, **"I used to drink a half-bottle to a full bottle of wine every night. Despite this delicious habit, I had to cut down because of the calories in wine. Depending on the wine, one glass of wine can range between 110—300 calories. The range has to do with alcohol content, inherent sweetness of the wine and serving size. I'm not advocating you only drink low calorie wine, but it never hurts to be familiar with the calorie count."**

Just today I went to a winery to talk with a friend who works there about a wine and cheese event. While waiting until she was free, I sipped a glass, full almost to the brim, of Vidal Blanc white wine, remembering that wines are 110-300 calories for a 6-ounce glass. I figured low end for this one. When I got home I looked up Vidal Blanc—50 calories per ounce. In actuality, the quantity served me was probably 8 ounces equal to 400 calories! And I don't really like wine!

Yes, I am aware of the research saying that a glass of red wine is good for your heart. So is a cup of grapes at 60 calories! Katherine Zeratsky, R.D., L.D., on the Mayo Clinic website, says, **"Some research suggests that whole grapes deliver the same amount of antioxidants that are in grape juice and wine but have the added benefit of providing dietary fiber."**

And ... and this is a big *and*, black coffee and tea are being found in more and more studies to be good for preventing various medical conditions such as heart disease and Parkinson's Disease—at 0 calories. My only warning would be to be aware of how sensitive you are to the caffeine in these beverages.

Another factor to consider before drinking beer and wine is that they stimulate your appetite. Can you drink a beer without munching on peanuts or pretzels? Or wine without cheese and crackers?

Can you stop with just one drink? I prefer to use most of my calories for things like grapes that include roughage (fiber), or drink 0-calorie A&W diet root beer (like a liquid dessert!), saving wine for special occasions.

Sharon Kay, M.A., L.U.T.

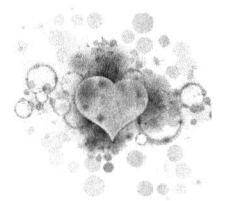

24: If You Bite It, Write It

The slogan "If you bite it, write it" is not original with me. I probably picked it up at Weight Watchers, but have heard it other places. It is a very valuable guide to controlling your dietary intake.

The number of calories that it is possible to consume simply tasting dishes that you are cooking is incredible. If you are in a workplace where cookies, candies and nuts are easily available, you can easily consume thousands of extra calories without even realizing that you are putting them in your mouth!

Unity teaches conscious awareness. What this means is simply becoming aware of all aspects of your personality, keeping the things you do that contribute positively to your well-being, and changing the things that don't.

I would refine the slogan even more by changing the order of the words to "If you write it, don't bite it." This means that pre-planning your meals and snacks, writing them in a ledger, and setting an intention of sticking to your plan makes it much less likely that you will binge eat from old habits which die hard.

Taking five minutes to write out your next day's meal plan may very well be the most important factor in learning to control your weight. It has been for me. It is not as difficult as it may sound. Most of us are creatures of habit and once you have a week or two of meals recorded you can easily go back and copy items that you are eating frequently. I do it in a form on my computer so it is simply a matter of copying and pasting. (See graph on page 200.)

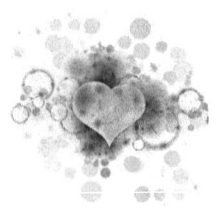

25: Learning to Listen to Your Body

Sometime in the 90s I developed a persistent metallic taste in my mouth. I researched online and discovered the possibility of a vitamin D deficiency. I began to take vitamin D capsules and the taste went away.

Today, if you do a search on Google for "metallic taste in mouth" you will find many alternate possibilities to consider. For me, at that time, it seemed easy enough to try taking vitamin D and, because it got rid of the taste, I decided that it was an accurate diagnosis.

Soon after moving to Unity Village in 2012, I saw a doctor for the purpose of establishing myself in the medical community. He ordered a standard blood profile and, though the metallic taste had never come back, it showed a vitamin D deficiency.

He explained that very few people, especially in northern states, get enough vitamin D. He calculated how much I would need and prescribed over-the-counter vitamin D which is very inexpensive. I have been taking 2000 I.U. per day ever since.

Our bodies talk to us constantly, giving us messages about what we need to do to maintain or improve our health. Very few of us listen. As you program yourself to eat quantities in line with achieving the weight that you want to be, you will feel lighter not just in your body but in your spirit as well. And you will be able to understand what your body is saying to you.

If you are feeling uncomfortable after a meal, you are probably not sick. Chances are very good that your body is telling you that you've eaten too much, eaten the wrong thing, or you are experiencing stress about something not related to food.

If I were to sit down right now and eat a 16-ounce steak, with all the trimmings, my body would react! The idea of processing all that

Sharon Kay, M.A., L.U.T.

fat, fiber and calories would overload my system. It is doubtful that I could actually force feed myself that much. Yet I did in the past.

The same is true with drinking large cups of fully–loaded strong coffee. You know the kind I'm talking about. The only way most people can stand coffee that strong is by diluting it with cream and sugar. Sugar- and fat-laden coffee, more appropriate as desserts, may very well be worse than frequent trips to vending machines when it comes to gaining or losing weight.

Within an hour of writing the above paragraph, I found myself with diarrhea! I went over my food diary from the previous day, considered what I had eaten, and saw there was nothing out of the ordinary or in excess quantity. Thus, based on what I had written, I had to assume that I had a virus.

Fortunately, it didn't last long, I didn't have any virus-type symptoms other than the diarrhea, and I was back to normal quickly.

Interestingly, I had weighed myself that morning. This is the first time since beginning this story that I have weighed on a day other than my Saturday weigh-in before the OA meeting. I have been taught that it is better to weigh only once a week, because our bodies fluctuate and getting on the scales can be traumatic if we feel that we have done well on our plan and they don't go down.

(**NOTE:** The next day's weigh-in was actually three pounds less. After the bout of diarrhea in the afternoon, I felt that this loss was "artificially inflated" by the release of extra fluids from my body so I chose to record the previous day's weight.)

My body had been talking to me all along.

One of my Unity teachers approached me one day as we were both about to get on an elevator. "The only reason I can say this to you," she said, "is because I have the same problem."

She proceeded to point out that I walked bent forward from the waist, a condition of which I was well aware. She suggested that 2 to 3 sessions with a chiropractor might be all it would take to correct the situation.

I felt it to my advantage to take the advice of a caring woman whom I felt had my best interests at heart. So I made some inquiries and five people recommended the same chiropractor. Going to him was a no-brainer.

His diagnosis? Weak muscles in the hip area for which he prescribed three exercises.

Within three weeks I was standing straight enough that my posterior protruded much less. I continue to go to the chiropractor for tweaking, and today I stand much straighter and taller and am proud of the way I look—though I am still a work in progress. I highly recommend chiropractic work if you have any spinal challenges.

A benefit to losing weight more slowly is that your skin has a chance to shrink back to a more normal state. If you are my age, you will never be 30 again. However, I believe you can restore your body to an age-appropriate radiance—a radiance that comes from inside as you learn to express your true beauty.

Can infirmities be healed by weight loss? I believe many can, but what I believe is not what heals you. When a woman touched the hem of Jesus' garment she was immediately healed. His words to her? "Daughter, thy faith hath made thee whole; go in peace, and be whole of thy plague." Mark 5:34 (KJV) Do you believe you can be healed by losing weight?

Losing 100-pounds in 1995/96 created a hernia in my body. Surgery to correct it threw my system into an imbalance which created ulcers in my bladder. I was diagnosed with Interstitial Cystitis which medical doctors consider incurable. Subsequent surgical procedures removed the ulcers, but I was left with what appeared to be limited bladder capacity

In 2015, as I released the remaining excess weight, I noticed that trips to the bathroom were becoming less and less frequent. Today I consider myself healed. Excess weight presses on our gastrointestinal areas and can create an illusion of serious physical conditions.

An even better example is my son who is now free of medications for numerous serious illnesses, all of which were corrected by losing weight. Yes, he used what I consider radical means to release the weight, but research shows that weight loss, regardless the method, can have a dramatic effect on a person's health.

All that is necessary is finding the motivation to lose the weight and finding the right weight loss plan for you.

You can do it! I believe in you!

Sharon Kay, M.A., L.U.T.

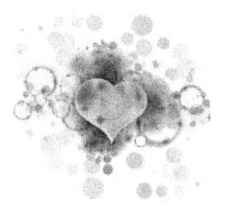

26: I Can't Be Perfect
All the Time

Even when you are highly motivated and well on the path to your goal weight, things happen. A little over two weeks ago I had oral surgery (considering that this is the third time I've mentioned this experience it obviously had a significant role in my psyche).

Even though I knew it was fairly major work I fully expected after the surgery to go home, take two powerful pain pills my dentist prescribed, get a really good night's sleep, and be right back to normal the next day. Not quite...!

The surgery included having an incision made in the roof of my mouth, scraping out a persistent infection from around a root canal, and cutting off the tip of the root. I was in the chair for over two hours.

I did get a good night's sleep that night, never felt serious pain, but over the next two weeks I felt very weak. It was difficult for me to make decisions, including planning meals, and true to my old patterns of behavior, I did not plan meals. I bought fast food much of the time and did not make good choices.

As a result, I gained five pounds.

Getting sick can throw our bodies out of sync. The major benefit of keeping track of what goes into your body is that you can more easily identify things that may be creating an out of balance situation.

I had no problem doing this. In addition to feeling weak, or low energy, my blood pressure was higher than normal. The latter is what caused me the most concerned. So I Googled (don't you love it!) for "10 ways to lower your blood pressure without medication" and found a list on www.MayoClinic.org, a website that I trust.

Going over the list I realized that my diet over the time I was healing from the surgery consisted of too much salt and too little potassium (which helps counteract sodium). I decided to buy some potassium tablets to increase my level.

Ordinarily, I prefer to get nutrients from food, but when our bodies are depleted of a vitamin or mineral it is often difficult to get the quantities we need from only the food we eat. I took just one 595mg. tablet a day for one week.

At the same time I went back to watching my salt intake. The next time I checked my blood it was back where it should be. At that point I went back to depending primarily on foods such as bananas, avocadoes and sweet potatoes which are all high in potassium.

My biggest motivator, however, is you! In the midst of writing this book I found myself having a problem staying on the weight loss plan that I had set for myself. I was going faithfully to an OA meeting and a weight loss group at work.

Yet there were about two months during which I had a very difficult time staying on track. What brought me back into focus was the knowledge that if this book didn't get written I would never have the opportunity to help you. I truly believe tools I am presenting in this book, combined with my personal experiences, will be powerful motivators for you.

As I continually reinforce, we create each other and I see you as the beautiful, creative god or goddess that you truly are. In doing so I know that I am the same.

Sharon Kay, M.A., L.U.T.

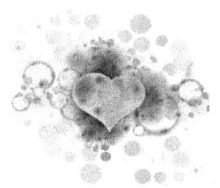

27: Taking a Break

In 1985, the first summer after entering college for the first time, I followed the Weight Watchers program and lost 75-pounds. You will read elsewhere how I gain that weight back when I divorced.

This is true; however, there were other factors at play. Most important, probably, is that I just wasn't ready emotionally to fully emerge from my shell of protection.

My body needed a break. Unfortunately, I had not learned how to maintain the loss (through no fault of Weight Watchers) and quickly regained the weight.

Ten years later, in 1995/96, I lost 100-pounds. I had learned more by this time, kept it off 12 years, and when the trauma of a second divorce occurred only gained half of it back.

Progress!

Again, however, I wasn't ready to face the real world of the slender woman and all that entails, including dating—something I was never very good at.

After moving to Unity Village, while taking classes, a professor videotaped each student doing a required oral presentation. I sounded fine—but I deplored the way I looked "on stage"!

It didn't take me long to lose about 35-pounds.

Then I took another break. I maintain most of that loss and, in January 2015, realized that it was time to release more weight.

Again, I took off about 25-pounds, followed by five months of unplanned maintenance.

Maintenance! A major milestone. I ate what I wanted, when I wanted and maintained the weight loss. This is my goal for myself and for you.

At the end of that five months I went back into weight loss mode and lost to my ultimate goal weight—a weight that is comfortable for me and at which I believe I look my best.

The point of this is that losing weight puts a different kind of stress on our systems—even a shock to the system. I believe that losing a set amount, for example 10% of your current weight, and planning to maintain that loss for a period of time is very healthy.

It gives our bodies a chance to feel the difference the lower weight makes, adjust to it, and mentally and emotionally change the way we think and act. In addition, it gives our skin as much opportunity as possible to shrink to the new size.

When I was 20, even 30, my skin was very elastic and it's amazing how much expansion/contraction it could endure and come out looking good even after dramatic weight loss. At age 67 gravity has taken more of a toll; yet, I am not unhappy with the way I look in clothes—naked is another story.

Sharon Kay, M.A., L.U.T.

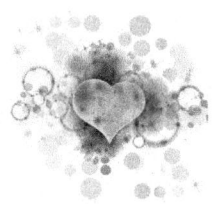

28: Let's Talk About Gas

You know the sound that is made when a chiropractor makes an adjustment... the sound made when people crack their knuckles... the sound made when you've eaten too many beans? Gas, or flatulence, plays an important role in the functioning of our bodies and improper diet can throw it out of balance.

Did you know that people who are lactose intolerant simply produce excess gas when they eat dairy products? That excess gas can be quite painful. My chiropractor suggested that I try avoiding dairy for a month, to test whether it was causing blood clots in my urine as an autoimmune reaction. I tried coconut milk first, reasoning that if coconut oil is good for me coconut milk should also be good for me, right?

Wrong! Within an hour I was having lactose intolerance symptoms. It took me about 48 hours to recognize that the only thing I had added to my diet was coconut milk. I changed to almond milk and the symptoms disappeared.

When you go to bed do you sleep well? Or do things like GERDS, gas or urinary frequency keep you from sleeping?

GERDS, an abbreviation for gastroesophageal reflux disease, is a chronic digestive disease. *GERDS* occurs when stomach acid or, occasionally, stomach content, flows back into your food pipe (esophagus).

My symptoms never got bad enough to consult a doctor, but 3-4 times a month I would go to bed and get up in the middle of the night with regurgitated acidity in my throat. This irritation was so bad that it took quite a while before I could go back to sleep. I treated it with over-the-counter antacids and would have to sleep sitting up with pillows propped behind my back.

Almost immediately after limiting my nighttime eating to a no later than 6 p.m. meal time the symptoms ceased to occur and have never returned.

I firmly believe that proper diet can cure almost any dis-ease. Notice the hyphen in the word disease. The founders of Unity taught that any medical problem is a result of our body not being at ease with itself. Thus, if we learn to listen to our bodies, we can put them back to a state of being at ease.

According to Michael F. Picco, M.D., of the Mayo Clinic GERD is a more advance stage of acid reflux. He says online that, **"If you have occasional acid reflux, lifestyle changes can help: Lose excess weight, eat smaller meals, and avoid foods that seem to trigger heartburn—such as fried or fatty foods, chocolate, and peppermint. Avoiding alcohol and nicotine may help, too."**

His recommendation: Treat acid reflux with over-the-counter medication unless your symptoms worsen.

In addition, many times what I thought was a urinary tract problem was actually a bowel problem. It is certainly not surprising considering everything I may have eaten just before going to bed.

Folks, our digestive systems are meant to be highly sophisticated processing plants. When we overload them, just as is true of mechanical parts in a factory, they go out or they cease to function at optimal capacity.

I spent many miserable nights which I now know were brought on by my own gluttony. It is alarming that gluttony is actually not listed as a sin in the Bible (though many think it is) because it is probably more harmful to us as individuals than some of the Ten Commandments.

Sharon Kay, M.A., L.U.T.

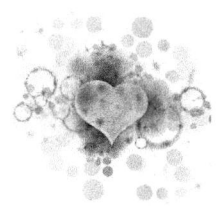

29: How Much Should I Weigh?

Several years ago, while living in Houston, Texas, I befriended a homeless man. He had some powerful spiritual gifts and I arranged for an in-home event that gave him some love offering spending money.

One day I took him to a fast food restaurant and the conversation of weight came up. He made the statement that I wasn't really that much overweight. I said, "How much do you think I weigh?"

He said a number... then said, "Oh wait ... I forgot to figure in the shelf!" Shelf? He was referring to the fact that my posterior protruded remarkably at the time. When he added 25-pounds to include that area, he was very close to correct.

So the question, "How much should I weigh?" varies dramatically for each individual and is probably not the number on standardized charts. I have been almost to the weight that insurance companies say I should be and, in my words, "I look like warmed over death!"

My desire is to look healthy. I recommend that you look at yourself naked in front of a mirror. Think to yourself, "I'd look pretty good if I lost 10... 25... 50-pounds." That then is your goal. When you reach that goal you don't have to stop losing if you don't want to. We're entitled to change our minds.

For the moment, however, your weight loss goal is 10 percent of your current weight. When you have lost 10 percent of your weight, no matter what the number is, you will feel great, have more energy and have a more positive outlook on life.

You were created as a unique individual by the God of your understanding and only trial and error can tell you what is good for your body and what isn't. But you can learn and you can establish a balance that is pleasing not only in appearance, but in the way your body feels.

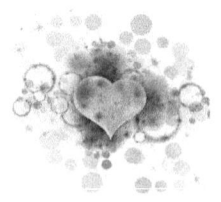

30: Hunger Pangs

At the present time I am releasing 1-2 pounds a week. I find my regimen to be quite easy for me to follow 95% of the time, but that does not mean that I never experience hunger pangs. Just today it seemed to take forever for my lunch break to come around.

So what do I do? Raid the vending machine? No!

So you lost "Only" One Pound?

THAT'S SOMETHING TO BE PROUD OF!

One of my tools is to visualize a pound of actual fat that has been removed from a human body. It is not a pretty sight (see photo at left). Then visualize the actual number of pounds that I am no longer carrying.

That is a lot of fat! In fact, if it were in a garbage bag and I tried to pick it up I would have to struggle do so. Yet, for years I carried it on my body.

And it is a lot of motivation to stay on my plan. At those times I tell myself that the hunger pangs are fat being dissolved.

But what about the times when visualization just doesn't work? As we age nutritionists tell us that it is better to eat several small meals a day than 1-3 large meals. I pack my weekday meals in a carrier to keep in the refrigerator at work. Sometimes my lunch needs to be divided into two meals—a 15 minute snack and a 30 minute meal. It satisfies me more than a candy bar from the vending machine would and I have consumed no more calories/points than I would have in eating the entire meal at one time.

My snacks are primarily fruit and I find that the sugar in fruit is very good at keeping hunger pangs at bay. And, due to the nature of my work (talking all day), I allow myself 2-3 natural throat lozenges which have the added benefit of a pleasant taste in my mouth which helps me to not think of food. Tic Tacs or gum would have the same effect and, for me, it does not have to be sugar free.

Sharon Kay, M.A., L.U.T.

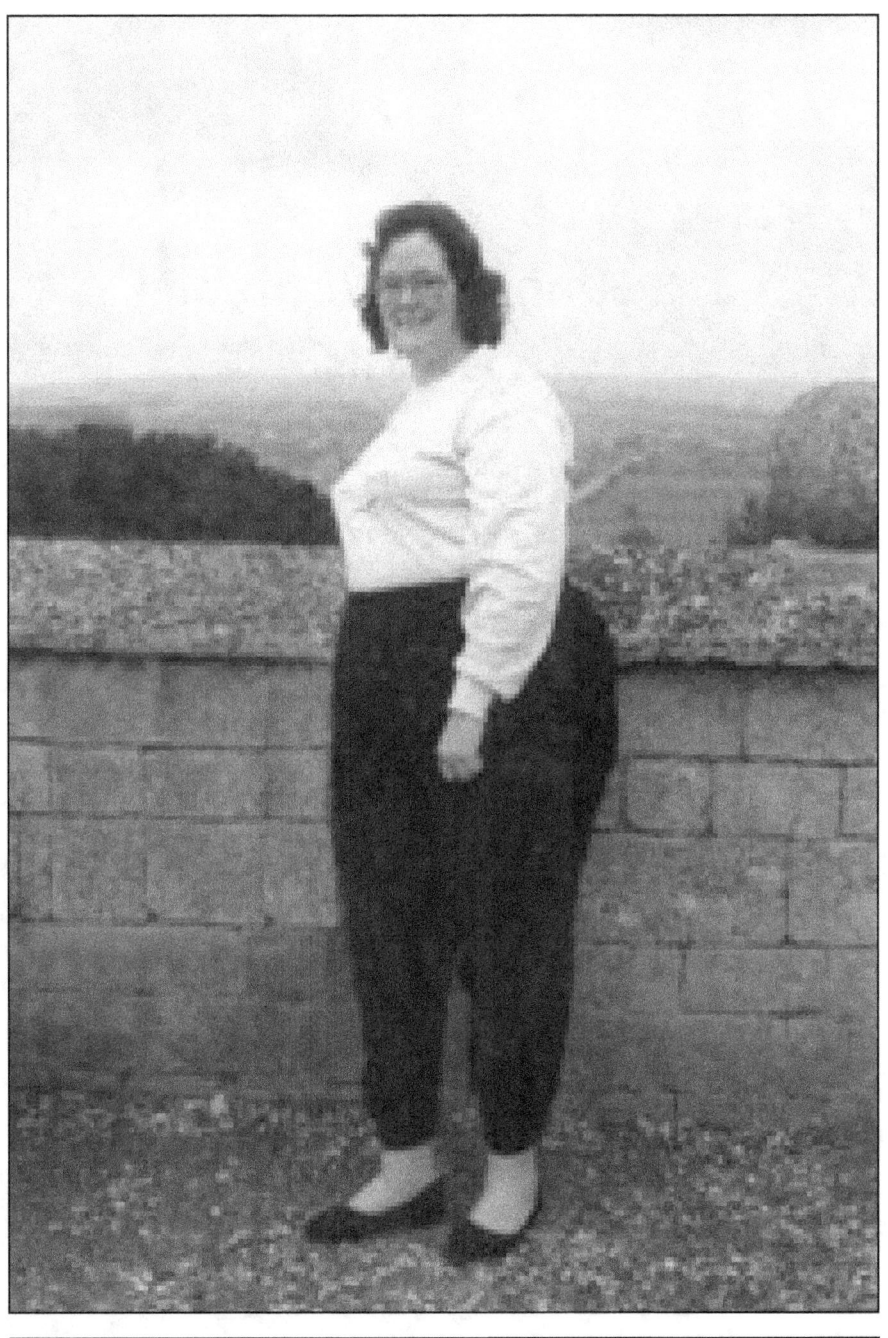

1992—Highest Weight of 296 1/2-pounds

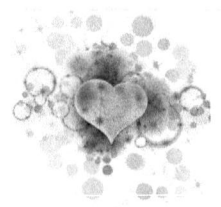

31: Preparing Yourself Physically

"Just lose weight and you'll be fine," the doctor said and walked out. Poor health and being overweight often go hand-in-hand. In 1996 my husband and I drove to Asheville, North Carolina. I ended up in an emergency room, my neck swollen as wide as my head. The only thing a doctor could suggest was an allergic reaction and prescribed an anti-histamine. Upon returning home I saw my personal doctor. I was at my highest weight—296 1/2-pounds (see photo on page 95) and his words, without doing any tests or exams, were painful for me to hear.

In spite of this, I had never had a diagnosis of high cholesterol, diabetes, heart problems, blood pressure requiring medication, etc. All my life I heard doctors say, "You are in perfect health ... just lose weight." Why couldn't they take me seriously?

I walked out of that office, never to return, swearing that no doctor would ever say that to me again. I drove in an almost straight line into a Weight Watchers meeting and proceeded to lose 100-pounds over a one-year period. Obviously his words, and my anger, motivated me at a deep level. (In hindsight, thank you doctor whose name I have forgotten.)

My husband was amazed at my steady weight loss. He said he had seen women gain weight - - but never intentionally, methodically, scientifically lose like I was losing. He had not thought it was possible.

This isn't surprising. In fact, many times weight gain is triggered by an upcoming marriage. The problem is that women starve them-selves before the wedding in order to get into a certain size dress. Stressors during preparations for marriage and the ceremony itself drive them back to their normal way of coping—eating.

The biggest problem with the vast majority of diets is that they encourage you—practically force you—to lose weight quickly. In doing so, while you may lose 30. 40. 50-pounds quickly, you compromise your health and weaken your body's resistance to illness. Stress, both at home and on the job, may feel even more overwhelming than usual.

What you are aiming for is good health, not a size 2 . 4 . 6 or a number on a chart. When I moved to Lees Summit, Missouri, I established myself with a holistic medical doctor. At my first visit he ordered a complete blood profile, recorded weight and blood pressure and we talked for a few minutes.

On my second visit we discussed the results of the lab work. Everything was well within normal limits. My weight was 50-pounds more than it is now. He did not consider that a major concern since everything else was normal. Blood pressure was slightly elevated which he attributed to:

- Stresses of a new job
- Seeing a new doctor for the first time
- A date that night with man I met on an online dating site

... enough to raise anyone's blood pressure!

Your numbers may not be as good as mine, but most numbers can be improved. The first thing I would do if I were working with you is analyze metaphysically any perceived health challenges. I say "perceived," because we create dis-ease in our bodies. No, of course we don't do it intentionally, but every time I've had a health challenge and could analyze it my personal "diagnosis" was mental or emotional issues.

These were often called psychosomatic illnesses (in your head) when I was a psychology student, but anyone who has ever felt pain of any kind, regarding whether the source is physical, mental, emotional or spiritual —knows that it hurts!

As a child, for example, I had strep throat every year! A week before my wedding, which took place on my 18th birthday, I had strep throat so bad that the doctor could not heal it out-patient and admitted me to the hospital. In hindsight, metaphysically, my body was screaming a message that I did not know how to interpret at that time.

Louise Hay attributes throat problems to "The inability to speak up for one's self. Swallowed anger. Stifled creativity. Refusal to change." With a sergeant mother in the position of power in my home this was, as our British friends say, "Spot on!" The marriage was an escape and, in reality, it served its purpose. My primary mistake was not getting out of it soon enough.

By analyzing our health challenges we can figure out what is going on mentally and emotionally that causes us to stuff ourselves with food just as we are stuffing our thoughts and emotions by not expressing them in a healthy manner. Too often, if you are like me and if you are reading this book I know that we have much in common, we force ourselves to stay in relationships for reasons that are not healthy.

Anything we have to force ourselves to do will ultimately result in failure. We have to recognize what psychologists call "secondary rewards" that we receive from those relationships and from being overweight. You know what I'm talking about. It is the things that get you attention.

Child psychologists recognize that many children act out (and are prescribed drugs for ADD or a variation) because of a need for attention they're not getting at home. Negative attention is better than no attention; thus, disruptive behaviors which result in punishment.

We do the same thing with our weight except that we've learned more skilled manipulation ... and don't think we don't use them.

Losing weight slowly, steadily, with even occasional breaks, provides a much safer approach to weight loss. At the same time we give ourselves opportunities to learn why we handle food as we do.

A serious medical challenge in 1996 interrupted my weight loss at almost exactly 100-pounds; however, in retrospect, I was a size 10/12 and at 5' 9" looked really good (see photo at left.) I have since realized that numbers on a doctor's office chart are not one-size-fits-all—in spite of what insurance companies would have you believe.

At the time my husband and I were building a successful international business, were traveling and bought a luxury sports car. Life was good and, in spite of the illness, I maintained the 100-pound loss for 12 years.

When marital challenges became more than I chose to endure I asked for a divorce and allowed the trauma/drama to drive me to my drug of addiction—food—and gained 50-pounds. I count that as success! During the last divorce drama I had gained back all that I had lost ... and more. Though it fluctuated, I maintained the 50-pound loss for another six years.

According to Hay, physical illnesses, including obesity, and other limitations stem from mental and emotional blockages. Charles Fillmore, co-founder of Unity, taught that thoughts, words spoken and actions taken create our world, including health challenges. And Mike

Dooley made famous the phrase, "Thoughts become things," through his "Notes from the Universe" (www.tut.com)

I believe it. And I have proven the principles to myself time after time since discovering these resources. For example, sometime during my second marriage I fell down a flight of stairs while sleepwalking—14 steps. Fortunately they were carpeted; however, I ended up with the entire right side of my body black and blue.

I woke up to my husband saying, "You know you don't have insurance. You don't need to go to an emergency room, do you?" (One of the reasons we're divorced.) So I didn't go. My wrist seemed mildly sprained, but healed uneventfully. The rest appeared to be superficial bruising and carpet burns, probably from sliding two-thirds of the way down. I don't remember the fall, nor did I feel any of the pain that must have put me into a state of shock. Of course, there is no doubt in my mind that SEVERAL of my angels rushed to cushion the fall.

About three months later I began to experience hip pain so severe that it was traumatic to get out of bed in the morning. I ended up sleeping on an air mattress on the floor. As long as I could crawl off the mattress and stand up slowly I was okay. A doctor attributed it to sciatic nerves, but with no insurance we couldn't afford treatments.

Hay's interpretation? Hip pain is said to stem from "Fear of, or inability to, move forward." This was so true of my marriage. I began affirming, "I move forward in life with ease and joy." Within a month the pain had decreased. Within three months it had disappeared entirely and it has never come back. Within a year I was divorced. Thoughts become things!

Previously, in trying to figure out why my bladder burned all the time, I had been diagnosed with hypothyroidism and prescribed medication. (Subsequently ulcers were found/Hay: Pissed off. Usually at the opposite sex. [laughter]) The medication didn't seem to make any difference, I felt that the doctor was clutching at a straw to give me something to focus on other than the bladder, I stopped taking the pills.

In the years between that first diagnosis and 2012 when I moved to Unity Village, whenever I had bloodwork done, the lab work showed low thyroid and medication was prescribed. Each time I would take a few tablets, decide I didn't believe the diagnosis (there were no symptoms other than a Thyroid Stimulating Hormone [TSH] number), and stop taking them.

(DO AS I SAY ... NOT AS I DID. DO NOT STOP TAKING PRESCRIPTION MEDICATION. IF YOU ARE NOT SUPPOSED TO BE TAKING IT, YOUR LABWORK WILL IMPROVE AFTER YOU START DOING THE AFFIRMATIONS.)

In January 2013 I went to a new doctor who ordered an extensive blood profile. Thyroid: NORMAL. A subsequent set of labs in 2014 showed the same results. No thyroid problem.

Hay on thyroid—"Humiliation. 'I never get to do what I want to do. When is it going to be my turn?'" Words I had said during my marriage came back to haunt me. "As long as I was willing to walk in his shoes I knew that I would go places and do things that I would never have dreamed that I would do." But his dreams were not my dreams.

Divorcing and subsequently moving to Unity Village was equivalent to taking charge of, and ultimately being responsible, for my own life.

By now are you ready to go out and buy Hay's book ... or take it off the shelf where it is gathering dust?

What does she say about being overweight? "Fear, need for protection. Running away from feelings. Insecurity, self-rejection. Seeking fulfillment." It all applied to me. What about you?

Don't misunderstand me. I go to doctors and value their expertise. Thankfully, many are becoming more holistic in their approach. If they can do something quickly, minimally invasively, without prescribing long-term prescription medications, and with high expectations of success, they act as instruments for healing. On the other hand, try working with Hay's affirmations if your symptoms elude diagnosis and you go from doctor to doctor looking for answers and relief from symptoms; or if doctors have called your condition "incurable." You have nothing to lose (except weight) and everything to gain in terms of restoring your health.

Myrtle Fillmore, co-founder of Unity Church of Christianity, healed herself of tuberculosis (which was considered incurable at the time) using prayer and affirmations. Her remarkable life story can be read in *Myrtle Fillmore: Mother of* Unity by Thomas E. Witherspoon, 1984.

She had been told by her family and by doctors that she had inherited the condition and was not expected to live past her 20s.

Witherspoon says that:

"By the spring of 1886, it appeared that the end of life for Myrtle Fillmore was near."

But in a service by Rev. E. B. Weeks, Myrtle heard the words "I am a child of God and therefore I do not inherit sickness."

Myrtle found that these words resonated for her as truth. She went home talking about the experience and began to talk lovingly to her body, claiming health and vitality for each and every organ and tissue.

Over a two year period she regained her strength and doctors could find no trace of the illness remaining in her system.

A one sentence synopsis of Myrtle's dynamic story is that she married Charles Fillmore in 1881, they had three sons, and she lived a long, happy life, dying in 1931 at age 86.

What do you need to heal?

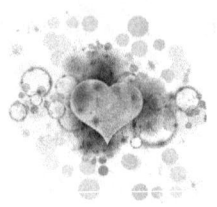

32: Diabetes

My mother was severely diabetic and both my children ended up with adult onset diabetes. Perhaps that means I was a carrier. Fortunately for me that means I have never had a high blood sugar reading and it is certainly not because I have watched my sugar intake.

I have been told by friends that some of the things I eat may not be diet-friendly for a diabetic. I understand the need for balancing blood sugar levels and that certain foods like white potatoes should be limited. Sweet potatoes or yams apparently do not cause as dramatic a spike in blood sugar levels. However, when I read a Glycemic Index chart it shows that a white potato has a "load" of 56 and a sweet potato is only slightly less at 54.

When interacting with diabetic friends I have observed that they often eat things that seem counterproductive ... but I will assume that they know what they're doing in this area better than I do.

As for me, though, most fruits are much lower on the Glycemic Index than other food items.

Sharon Kay, M.A., L.U.T.

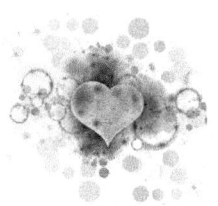

33: Sensitivities
and Allergies

My personal chart tracking my weight loss shows that during the month of June I had a large weight gain. This reflects two things: 1) I am human just like you; and 2) our bodies are capable of giving the appearance of putting on weight seemingly overnight.

In that instance I had had about six weeks of not staying on my plan well following oral surgery, but the surgery was just an excuse. The final weekend of that binge culminated in a friend's family reunion.

I didn't go prepared and the buffet consisted of fried chicken, coleslaw dripping in mayonnaise, potato salad, yeast rolls, and lots of desserts. There wasn't much other than some fresh tomatoes that would have been on my plan.

AUTOIMMUNE DISORDERS

It was very easy to say, " I'll get back on plan tomorrow." And I did. But not before I spent a horrible night. The silver lining to the cloud is that I was able to put together some bits and pieces of medical information that I had gleaned over the years and recognized that I have an autoimmune condition which causes my eliminatory organs to swell when I eat foods that they don't like.

The drive home was miserable but, fortunately, I was travelling with a woman who understood the need for frequent bathroom stops. To put it delicately, it is very difficult for our bodies to release waste matter when our internal organs are swollen. At time such as this I am only able to release about a tablespoonful of urine each time we stop.

When I got home I immediately went back to following my plan, but I also included some testing to determine what I was putting in my body that was causing the reactions I was having.

I use a pendulum, in much the same way that people used to do water witching to find water, to test whether something will adversely affect my body. (Yes, I already knew this technique. Why hadn't I already been doing it?) I simply hold a pendulum near a food and ask the question, "Will this food cause an autoimmune reaction in my body?"

I know this will sound "woo woo" to many of you, but there is much scientific evidence to support its validity.

The first food rejected was, believe it or not, watermelon. We were nearing July 4th and everyone knows that watermelon is a favorite for that holiday. I had a big one in my refrigerator and Weight Watchers tells us that we can eat all the fruit we want without causing weight gain.

So I cut a large slice and tested it. The more harmful a food is for your body, the bigger the arc of the pendulum. My pendulum went wild!

Now, lest you think that I am looney and immediately stop reading this book, I went to the internet and Googled why watermelon might be detrimental to my body. I found the following quote:

"This summer treat is sweet and refreshing, but it could be the sneaky cause of stomach bloat. Watermelon is high in fructose, a naturally occurring sugar that is often incompletely absorbed by our GI system, leading to gas. Experts estimate one in three people suffer from fructose malabsorption." Liz Vaccariello from *21-Day Tummy* (Reader's Digest Association Books)

Similar symptoms may occur if a person is lactose intolerant (dairy). According to www.mayoclinic.org, "The signs and symptoms of lactose intolerance usually begin 30 minutes to two hours after eating or drinking foods that contain lactose. Common signs and symptoms may include: diarrhea, nausea and vomiting, abdominal cramps, bloating, gas."

My primary symptom has always been gas, but there have been times of abdominal cramping, especially when I was pregnant with my two children. (I remember a time during my first pregnancy when double dating with another couple that I ran everyone out of the car! I'll leave it to you to imagine why!)

The week following making this discovery and getting back on my dietary plan the excess weight caused by bloating and fluid retention (internal, not external) released easily and I dropped all of the weight in one week. This is also reflected on the chart.

Sharon Kay, M.A., L.U.T.

WHEAT

When my bladder was so bad I was seeing urologist, neurologist, gynecologist, allergist, et al, and spent thousands of dollars in doing so. In spite of extensive testing, the allergist did not find anything that should be causing the bladder pain.

In reading the book *Wheat Belly* by William Davis, M. D. (2011), however, I realized that sensitivity, as opposed to an allergy, might be having an effect. In addition, he explained that wheat acts like a narcotic in our brains and this made total sense to me. I have been wheat-free much of the time since reading the book.

I found that within a week of avoiding wheat products, before I had lost pounds, my abdominal area had gone down extensively. It is a really good start to a weight loss program, and I've also noticed that as long as I avoid wheat there are two other advantages: 1) I look and feel better; and 2) I find that bakery products, including the seductive aroma of fresh baked goods at a grocery store, do not tempt me to buy them.

According to Dr. Davis:

"... today's wheat has been genetically altered to provide processed-food manufacturers the greatest yield at the lowest cost; consequently, this once benign grain has been transformed into a nutritionally bankrupt yet ubiquitous ingredient that causes blood sugar to spike more rapidly than eating pure table sugar and has addictive properties that cause us to ride a roller coaster of hunger, overeating, and fatigue."

DAIRY

I mentioned to my chiropractor that I occasionally have blood clots in my urine which are not associated with infection. He said, "No, they are an autoimmune reaction. I would suspect dairy products. Try avoiding dairy for a month and see what happens."

I did. Voila! No blood clots! Today I use only almond milk, use cheese sparingly, and find that I feel much better when I avoid dairy.

You will call that I first tried substituting coconut milk for cows' milk and had not just a sensitivity reaction, but a full-blown allergic reaction. Fortunately, because I knew what I was putting into my body, it didn't take me long to identify the culprit. When I changed to almond milk my body returned to balance.

You would probably not have the same effect, but this situation illustrates how important it is to know what we're ingesting.

SALT

Recently I went to my chiropractor for a regularly scheduled appointment. I had lost weight, was feeling really good, and it had been several appointments since they had taken my blood pressure and weight. So I figured it was a good time to check my blood pressure and asked the assistant to do it.

On the first try my blood pressure was extremely high. Same for the second try. A different cuff yielded a much lower result, but it was still higher than it should be.

The doctor and I discussed other variables, because he had checked my ankles and there was no swelling and I was calm with no upsets. We focused on the fact that I was not limiting salt intake and I decided to give that a try because I'm opposed to taking medications.

Two days later I noticed that I was feeling weak, had mild stomach cramps, and nothing in my diet should have caused these symptoms. I considered the fact that I had stopped adding salt to my food, though I had not gone totally salt free.

I was amazed to find the following information by Googling:

"Salt is a chemical compound consisting of sodium, which is detrimental to health. When a person drastically restricts his intake of salt for an extended period of time, the old accumulations in the body are excreted through the skin and kidneys.

"Withdrawal symptoms: In the initial days, there may be a salty taste in the mouth. "Cramps are initially experienced as salt is removed from the diet or rapidly excreted from the body," adds Honey Khanna, nutritionist at MaxHealthcare. Other withdrawal symptoms include high blood pressure, lethargy and drowsiness, and excessive urination [as salt is water retentive]. In extreme cases, you may experience hypernatremia [electrolyte disturbance in the body] and fits.

"Cure: Reduce salt intake slowly. Replace regular salt with rock salt or low-sodium salt." (http://completewellbeing.com/article/parting-pangs/)

While this website considers salt to be an addictive substance, I would consider it to be something that I am sensitive to—and I'm not sure there's much difference. One school of thought for alcoholism says that alcoholics are highly sensitive to alcohol; thus, the craving leads them to excess.

What sensitivities or allergies may be abetting your obesity?

Sharon Kay, M.A., L.U.T.

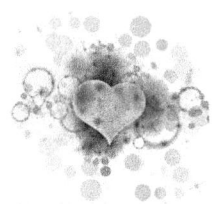

34: Forget About Exercising
... You Won't Do It Anyway

The young, slender, athletic doctor, male or female, says to John or Jane Doe, "I don't want you to start out exercising strenuously. Just get out and walk around the block. Increase the distance a little bit each day and soon you'll be out jogging with me." They mean it as motivation to approach losing weight and getting fit slowly and easily.

"Okay," you mumble under your breath knowing full well how much it hurts to just walk from your car into the grocery store. Your back hurts ... your inner thighs, especially in the summer, chafe and burn. "Just walk," you tell yourself and stop on the way home at a drive-thru for a hamburger, fries and sugar-laden supersized soft drink.

When I lost 75-pounds in the 1980s I pretty much stayed in bed or on the sofa watching television through the first 20-pounds. I simply followed the Weight Watchers program of the time which was *very* rigid—and allowed my body to adjust to the lowered calorie intake. My energy level was so low that I needed to. As I started to feel better I began to move more.

I started with attempts to walk around the block. It was a long block and at first I couldn't do it. So I walked as far as I felt comfortable walking; then turned around and walked home. Gradually the distance increased.

Then I got a bicycle. I began exploring our neighborhood by bicycle and found that I enjoyed riding.

I joined a gym where I met a girlfriend 2-3 times a week. We worked out, then relaxed in the swimming pool and sauna. (Obviously, I was a stay-at-home mom at the time.)

At some point I decided to try riding the bicycle to the gym—five miles one way. I found I could do it and I did.

The woman you see in the photo on page 2 is the result. But, as you know from what I have said, it didn't happen overnight. It began by allowing my body to adjust slowly (in bed much of the time!) and to feel better before I expected to move like an athlete.

Oh, yes ... when I went back to college in the fall, I found that bowling was an option for a physical education credit. I was old enough that I could have opted out of PE, but I had bowled with my husband, was pretty good, even had my own special ball (clear polyurethane with a yellow rose embedded) and signed up. With the instruction of a professor whom I, frankly, had a crush on, I did quite well in the class.

Don't let anyone try to guilt or scare you into going full speed ahead into exercising when you first start losing weight. Move at your own pace. Your body will tell you when you are ready.

Also, don't ever think you have to enjoy the type of exercising that your friends enjoy. (Of course, if you want to remain friends with someone who loves to hike, you may want to take up hiking.) Don't try to force yourself to do something that is entirely foreign to your personality—unless it's something you've been waiting all your life to do.

There are some things on my "bucket list" that I either did not have the opportunity to do or felt that I was too heavy to be good at ... or then there's fear of failure. Look back at times in your life that you've tried something new. How many times have you been an utter failure? Maybe you didn't become a professional, but I doubt that you failed.

Is it time to try?

Just STOP the insanity of forcing yourself. Focus on one thing at a time. Focus on losing a few pounds. Five-percent of your current weight is a good number to aim for. Five-percent of my 250-pound was 12 1/2-pounds. By the time I reached that, in about one month, I actually felt like moving more. I began taking a longer walk to the bathroom for what my workplace calls "comfort breaks" about once an hour. I began taking one flight of stairs, up and down, once a day during my work week and I have stairs at home which I began to use more often.

You have my personal guarantee that the more you lose, the more you will feel like moving your body—and isn't that really all exercise is? In the meantime, do stretches when you are standing or sitting. When I'm waiting by myself to go into a meeting I bend backwards as far as I can comfortably, then forward, then side-to-side, holding each stretch for a few seconds.

Without noticeably "exercising," (Remember my affirmation in the Introduction?) I went down two pant sizes with my first 20-pounds.

While D I E T may be a 4-letter curse word, E X E R C I S E is another word that has negative connotations. For me it brings back memories of:

1) drill sergeant type physical education coaches (female as well as male) who were hired by school districts to force us to break out a sweat in the interest of controlling teenage hormones. Having to undress and show off my over-developed teenage body was worse than any horror movie. Being the last person to be chosen for any sport (until my school got a swimming pool and I was pretty good at water sports [since fat floats!]) left a lasting dislike of any form of sport, including most spectator sports.

2) skinny instructors in leotards that left nothing to the imagination doing calisthenics in exercise clubs and expecting my size 22+ body to keep up with them. Sex may sell, but I knew I would never look like they did—even if I were at goal weight. All I came out of those classes with was discouragement.

Fast forward to today. Replace the eight letters in exercise with M O V E M O R E. To emphasize what I said above, as I released weight:

- I found myself parking further from the door of the grocery store;

- I began walking up and down one flight of stairs at work instead of taking the elevator;

- I walked more at the grocery store than I needed to;

- I did stretches while I waited for my turn in our prayer chapel (part of my job)

- I did stretches at my desk designed to loosen joints that hadn't been used in a long time and any other movement I felt led to incorporate.

As you will read elsewhere in this book, I go to a chiropractor once a month. After seeing him for spinal alignment and being given three exercises for hip muscles which cranked me up to a standing position (as opposed to walking bent forward at the hips like an elderly bag lady!) I became convinced in the value of regular adjustments. He has worked miracles in my body and how I carry myself—rather like going to one of the finishing schools I used to see in movies where they would have young women walk around with books on their heads.

It is a tremendous thrill for me now to be able to sit with my legs crossed at the knees and one leg hanging down beside the other as opposed to sitting masculine style with an ankle on my thigh which was the best I could do with fatty thighs. In addition, thanks to my weight loss, I frequently cross one leg over the other and gently pull my foot toward my hip joint while pushing down on my knee to get in some good stretching.

Exercise does not have to be strenuous or involve repetitive counting (i.e. three sets of 10). Any movement that you can comfortable add to your daily routine will be beneficial. One of the most effective ways to move, recommended by all medical professions, is simply walking. I say "simply," but I know that it can be painful and not so simple when your inner thighs rub together until they're red and raw. That's one of the reasons I do extra walking in large grocery stores where there is air-conditioning. An air-conditioned indoor mall would also work and has an added advantage of providing places to sit when necessary.

In the beginning, just do your best. More opportunities for increased movement will be presented to you as the weight melts away.

If you are in a wheelchair or for some other reason cannot do any extra movement this next statement may seem strange, but it is used by athletes and physical therapists because it has been shown to be effective. Use the power of your mind to visualize yourself moving.

As Myrtle Fillmore discovered and taught, each of us has the power to overcome physical challenges. I affirm complete and total healing on all levels of your being.

NOTE: If your doctor has you doing any exercises for a specific condition do not stop because I said to! Before I began the Shape Shifting program my chiropractor had me doing three exercises for my back so that I would stand up straight. I did not stop doing those and the benefits were remarkable and very noticeable.

Sharon Kay, M.A., L.U.T.

After reading this section I am convinced that I can _____

_____

_____

_____

_____

_____

_____

_____

_____

_____

_____

_____

_____

_____

_____

_____

_____

_____

_____

_____

_____

_____

_____

_____

_____

PART FIVE

What Are

Your

Spiritual Issues?

SPIRITUAL ISSUES

My spiritual path has taken so many twists and turns that if you were looking at it from an aerial view it would look like a drunken snake had laid out my path!

I have come to understand, however, that there is no one right path and I had to explore many avenues before I had the experience many people talk about at Unity of "coming home."

I understand now, too, that I could have found it in any church home, any denomination, any spiritually oriented group. A friend in Texas is a high level leader in the Catholic Church. Yet when I talk with him it feels as though I'm talking Unity. We discussed this one day and he explained that there are many levels of faith in the Catholic Church. When he and I were talking we were talking on the mystical level of Catholicism. Since that conversation I have read that there are mystical branches of nearly every mainstream church.

There is a story of a woman who goes into a town expecting to find it difficult to find a job, people who will abuse her and no friends. She finds exactly what she was expecting to find. A second woman goes into the same town expecting to be successful and richly rewarded and to find loving people who will be kind to her and accept her as a friend. Guess what she found? Both women went to the same town, but their attitudes and expectations were different.

In spirituality, as in all walks of life, we find what we expect.

So how does this apply to weight loss? On the most basic level of our existence, at this point in time it would be called the quantum level, we are one with everything. If I truly believe that I was born to be happy, to be beautiful, to be wealthy, to be rewarded with fulfilling relationships I will create those things in my life through the energy I invest in certain areas.

If you truly believe that inside your obese body is a thin man or woman struggling to come out you will do everything within your power to chip away the excess layers of fat and set that person free. That is spirituality at its core essence. Dare I say that is salvation—saving ourselves from ourselves.

At one time I was taught that the order of the universe says that I am to put God first, others second, self last. That is so wrong! If we do not put ourselves, our health and well-being first we will die without ever truly having helped another person, much less ever being truly devoted to the God of our understanding.

Sharon Kay, M.A., L.U.T.

If we do not take care of ourselves and our needs, our tendency is to complain. We never have enough. Someone else is always to blame for the perceived lack in our life. In short, we are miserable. And, if we are miserable, and talk about it, why on earth would anyone else want to be like us?

I am a spiritual leader in my church; yet this was the hardest section for me to write. Why? I suspect it is because there are so many "brands" of spirituality. What you have read, and will continue to read in this book, is what I call "spirituality as opposed to religion." I grew up in a church that is heavy on doctrine. When I got to an age of being able to think rationally I realized that I could not believe in a punishing God. The more I studied the more I realized that a God who would punish us is a man made God created by males in a 325 A.D. meeting called the Council of Nicea.

These rulers of the time effectively took power away from people like you and me, especially women, and put it in the hands of the church. But don't take my word for it. Go to any theological research center and read about the Council of Nicea. If you grew up as I did it will be a revelation to you that so much of what we were taught is of human making, not God's Divine Plan for humankind.

My beliefs today are based on the teachings of Jesus the Christ who taught only love:

"Love one another as I have loved you." John 13:34 (KJV)

"Greater love hath no man than this, that a man lay down his life for his friends." John 15:13 (KJV)

"And now these three remain: faith, hope and love. But the greatest of these is love." I Corinthians 13:13 (NIV)

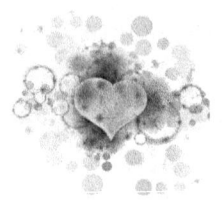

35: The Value of Forgiveness

If your issues are similar to those that follow, you are going to have to do a lot of forgiveness work—both of others and yourself—before you can move on to a healthy, happy lifestyle. I highly recommend the book *Radical Forgiveness* by Colin Tipping. It changed the way I looked at personal "abusive" situations and reminded me of one of my favorite Shakespearean quotes, "All the world's a stage, and all the men and women merely players ...."

Others

After spending seven years working on a master's degree in psychology and six years working on my certification to be a Licensed Unity Teacher, both of which require intensive soul searching, I felt that I had truly forgiven and/or made amends in all situations where forgiveness was required.

Imagine my surprise when an attorney called me wanting information to use against my former husband—and I found myself wanting to help the attorney and her client!

After working through my present day morals regarding this issue, I decided to do nothing unless I heard from the attorney. While I did not like the idea that my former husband had cheated a customer in ways that I observed while working with him, I no longer felt any animosity.

We had gone through a nasty divorce, during which he took away my access to money and hired a $400 per hour attorney to attack my integrity.

The turning point in my forgiveness was when I recognized that his being so nasty to me was necessary for my growth. If he had lived up to our verbal agreements and kept the promises he made, I would at this point be giving him credit for things that, in actuality, I and the God of my understanding deserve credit for as co-creators.

Sharon Kay, M.A., L.U.T.

Today I would go to my former husband and thank him, but unless his consciousness level has increased he would not understand. It is better for both of us to continue to follow our own paths.

Self

The most important person we have to forgive, however, before we can effectively release any addiction, is ourselves. It has always been easy for me to look back at my past and wallow in self-pity at the "woulda shoulda coulda dones."

"I should have found a way to go to college after high school instead of getting married at age 18." "I would have kept the weight off if I had married the right men and not felt that divorce was my only choice." "I could have had a successful career if I hadn't gotten pregnant." Notice that there is an element in each instance of blaming someone else rather than taking responsibility for my own choices.

One of the most powerful books that I have read is Eckhart Tolle's previously mentioned *The Power of Now*. One of the many things Tolle says which impacted me is that:

"Your mind is an instrument, a tool. It is there to be used for a specific task, and when the task is completed, you lay it down.

"As it is, I would say about 80 to 90 percent of most people's thinking is not only repetitive and useless, but because of its dysfunctional and often negative nature, much of it is also harmful. Observe your mind and you will find this to be true. It causes a serious leakage of vital energy.

"This kind of compulsive thinking is actually an addiction. What characterizes an addiction? Quite simply this: you no longer feel that you have the choice to stop. It seems stronger than you. It also gives you a false sense of pleasure, pleasure that invariably turns into pain."

Can you relate these words to your eating? I can. Compulsive thinking/compulsive eating. Doing anything without regard to the consequences is harmful on one or more levels. Even if you do not appear to be hurting yourself or anyone else on the physical realm, acting compulsively erodes us mentally and emotionally.

Today I do my best to simply enjoy the moment that I'm experiencing—the moment that the universe has promised me. I have no assurance that I will not have a heart attack or be hit by a car tomorrow, but in this moment I am safe in my home, healthy and happy. What more can one woman ask for?

Well ... I'm waiting for my twin flame to manifest. He will appear the minute that I totally embrace the woman that I am meant to be. Liking the woman I see in the mirror, liking the words I hear coming out of my mouth, liking all aspects of myself on all levels of being—physical, mental, emotional, spiritual.

What are you waiting for? There's no magic pill or potion. No knight in shining armor to rescue you from yourself. But you have the power to generate the creative energy you need to manifest anything you can imagine. You think you don't have enough strength (power) to raise yourself up from whatever depth you've sunk to; whereas, in reality, you are the only one who has the power.

Will you wield your power wisely or continue to waste your energy going in circles of "poor pitiful me"? If you spent half as much time being creative as you do feeling sorry for yourself you could have anything you wanted.

There, I've thrown down the gauntlet. In the past the term meant to challenge someone to a duel, but the only weapon I'm armed with is love. I love each and every one of you and I'm challenging you to put your past behind you and walk with me into a future so beautiful it is difficult to picture.

In 2008 I wrote an article I titled "Life at Age 1000." The logic behind the writing was that most people look at their predecessors, or at health challenges, and put a year on their tombstone—long before they're in a casket.

My mother had severe diabetes and did not attempt to take care of herself. In fact, she was in denial, refusing to admit that her sugar was out of control, stealing other residents' desserts after she had to be admitted to a nursing home. She died at age 65, in her sleep, from fluid around her heart.

It would have been so easy for me to put 2013 on my tombstone, but a wonderful doctor said to me, "You won't die young. You have too much living to do." Today, at age 67 I'm planning on another 20 years of working full-time and, frankly, I'll probably start another career after that. I have observed that retiring is pretty much a guarantee that death is just around the corner unless one stays active physically, mentally, and spiritually.

In the article, I challenged people to think about what they would change about their lives if they knew they were going to live to be 1000! That still seems far-fetched to most people and, if you can't begin to imagine that as a possibility, just add 20 years to your current set "death year."

Sharon Kay, M.A., L.U.T.

With modern medicine and surgical procedures, with body parts being grown from our own cells, it is not that much of a stretch to imagine living to 100 . 110 . 120.

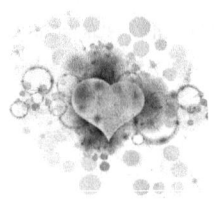

36: Fasting

In the late 1970s I felt led to do a 40-day fast. Having come from a Baptist background, where fasting was not practiced, It was a strange concept for me and I did not get support from family and friends. Doing the fast, however, became paramount in my thoughts.

I worked for a Methodist minister at the time and he agreed to monitor me for any mental changes that he might observe. A friend who was Pentecostal and a registered nurse agreed to meet with me regularly to monitor my vital signs.

Though my Baptist minister and my husband were disapproving, they recognized my need to do the fast and gave their approval as long as I agreed to stop if the Methodist minister or the nurse felt the fast was harming me.

It was one of the most amazing experiences of my life and led to dramatic changes. In the context of the book, though, weight loss was not one of them. Fasting has its place and I received many spiritual messages that were guidance for my future path, but I would never recommend it for weight loss.

Yes, I did lose about 40-pounds during that 40 days, and I felt fine the entire time, but it was because, as the scriptures say Jesus said, "I have meat to eat that ye know not of" (John 4:32 KJV). I was sustained by my faith during the fast.

After the period of fasting was over, and I gradually began to increase my dietary intake under the supervision of the nurse, the weight began to return and I ended up weighing more after the fast than I did before.

You see, I had learned nothing about safely releasing weight and keeping it off. I had learned more about how the God of my understanding works in my life, but the purpose of this fast was not to lose weight. It was for spiritual guidance.

Years following the fast seemed anything but spiritual. I found myself with a yearning to go to college for the first time. I had married

Sharon Kay, M.A., L.U.T.

almost straight out of high school, reared two children, and now it was time for mama's education. That didn't set well with a husband who had a G.E.D. from the Army.

"Your mother just wants to go to school and find another husband," my children were told repeatedly.

During the fast I dreamt of climbing a mountain. I would take 2-3 steps forward; then slide back a step. I persevered until I reached the top. Up to that point everything had been in black and white. When I stepped onto the plateau the vista changed to beautiful technicolor.

My college days seemed to validate the dream—2-3 steps forward; then back a step. The biggest slide came when I learned that my husband was a pedophile who had been molesting our daughter. It took over a year of his verbal abuse before I had the strength and courage to move out of that marriage and put myself through my M.A. while working full-time for a wonderfully supportive psychiatrist.

I got the answers I needed in order to move out of an abusive relationship by fasting. Would I do it again? Yes, if I felt the same spiritual guidance. Fasting is not, however, in my opinion, the answer for weight loss.

Yes, I lost weight, about a pound a day, while fasting. Those pounds, in spite of my best intentions, found their way back onto my body quickly. And fasting for other than spiritual purposes is not healthy.

One of my Dream Team editors debated the issue with me, citing the number of doctors and alternative medicine specialists who recommend fasting. She went on to say that, "I fast for 3-10 days at least once a year ... I do so to give my organs a rest and to cleanse them, but I follow the doctor's guidelines. I don't do it on my own."

I whole heartedly endorse her fast, but note the difference. I would call this a spiritual fast for cleansing and purifying the body. It is definitely NOT a fast to lose weight which is the topic of this book.

According to Jill Coleman, M.S., C.P.T., in a Feb. 7, 2014 "Prevention" magazine article entitled "The Scale Won't Move—Now What?" we may sometimes get stuck in our weight loss efforts where it seems impossible to lose weight no matter how hard we try. That is called a "set-point" and is a time when we may be tempted to fast the weight off.

Coleman says, **"The solution is to stop traditional dieting and extreme exercise approaches altogether, and find a way to eat and exercise you can do forever.**

"I recommend starting with nutritional changes only. Increase dietary protein and up your fibrous veggies (all veggies except starchy varieties like potatoes, corn, peas, etc.)

"Kick the sugar and booze.

"And then keep doing these things.

"Consistency with a tight nutrition plan is the most tried-and-true approach to resetting your weight. Consistency means not days or weeks, but months and years. The leanest people are the most consistent. They are not constantly trying new "diets" and meal plans—they find what works for them and stay 90% consistent 100% of the time with it."

If, however, you decide that fasting is the only way you can lose weight please don't try it without medical help.

Although I occasionally use the term "lose weight," I encourage you to erase the word "lose or lost" from your vocabulary. Whenever we lose something the idea is that it can, and should, be found. A much more positive approach is to "release" weight—allow it to move into the ethers and be found by a person who needs to gain weight.

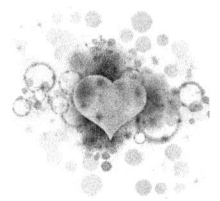

37: Releasing Negativity

My mother, who was a sergeant in the Women's Army Corp when she became pregnant with me, gave an appearance of being a no nonsense, gruff, negative to the extreme, woman. There were no hugs; no "I love you's" spoken in our home. Although I remember only one spanking while growing up, she disciplined through intimidation.

Combine this with the church's intimidation of going to hell for sins committed with the "Thou Shalt Nots" and I was surrounded by negativity. About all I could do without getting in trouble was study, go to church—or eat!

Early in my life I learned to counteract Mother's negativity by hiding behind interesting adventure books, which gave me a positive perspective. The negative energy, however, carried forward into two marriages. In regard to the first marriage, I recall the adage of a woman marrying a man "just like dear old dad." There was no male energy in our home so I married a man "just like dear old mom."

It wasn't until I discovered Unity's teachings of love, peace and joy that I reclaimed my personal power and was able to release that deeply entrenched negativity.

When I moved from Texas to Missouri it felt as though changing my latitude and longitude had moved me out of a negative energy field. In reality, I expected to find love, peace and joy at Unity Village and, just as with weight loss, we get what we expect. It wasn't the geography that was holding me back. It was my attitude.

Do any of you need to join me in an attitude adjustment?

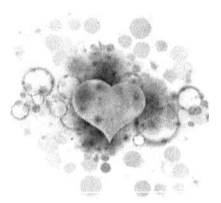

38: Attitude of Gratitude

This chapter title isn't original with me. I learned it through Unity and Unity probably borrowed it from some other tradition. Regardless the source, it is one of the most powerful concepts we can turn to whether we are committed to weight loss or any other physical, mental, emotional or spiritual challenge.

One of the most powerful prayers we can say is simply, "Thank you God. Thank you God. Thank you God." This works for individuals involved in their Christian and Jewish faiths, but what about the person who has given up on traditional religious practices? Even atheists believe in something. If it is more comfortable for you to simple believe in your own talents and abilities that works, too. Just change the words to "Thank you Sharon. (replace my name with your own). Thank you Sharon. Thank you Sharon."

I am grateful every moment of every day for the life that I have created for myself at Unity Village. I awaken every morning with the words "Thank you" coming from my heart and out of my mouth. It is so easy.

And, lest you think it's easy because my life is easy, remember that as I write these words I am a single woman, making less than $12 an hour, drive a 2001 car in 2015, and at this moment am waiting until next week's paycheck to be able to afford to create with my own hands the website that you can now go to at www.SharonKays.website.

So ... how can I be grateful? Well, why not?

1) I woke up this morning and my entire body was hurting.

3) I went to the bathroom and everything was functioning properly (as you've read elsewhere in the book that has not always been true and I am very grateful every time I can urinate without pain).

4) I had food in the apartment for today's meals and enough to last until the next paycheck,

5) I had more than enough gas in my car to last until payday.

6) I have three evening meetings to go to between now and payday where I will socialize with people who love (even better "like") me, knowing that any one of those people would loan me money if I had an emergency—but I won't. We create most of our emergencies by worrying about "what ifs" and I refuse to worry.

This is not to say that I do not plan. I have a retirement fund through work and put 15% of my before taxes income into that fund. My company contributes an additional 5%; thus, I am saving 20% of my income—and I won't touch it.

Even more important as an investment is that I tithe 14% of my gross income, time and talents to my church. I tip servers much more than 20% (unless the service is absolutely horrible which is seldom the case). And I donate to other charitable causes when my spirit guides me to do so.

If you don't attend a church, that doesn't exempt you from the Law of Reciprocity. What you give has to come back to you—though you have to develop eyes to see that the blessings are not always returned in the same way you gave.

I bet you didn't know that there are Universal Laws that govern every aspect of our lives. You can read more about them at:

http://www.abundance-and-happiness.com/universal-laws.html

"Universal Laws, also referred to as Spiritual Laws or Laws Of Nature," the website says, "are the unwavering and unchanging principles that govern every aspect of the universe and are the means by which our world and the entire cosmos continues to exist, thrive and expand. "

I'm not going to try to persuade you to believe the way I believe. If, however, this idea intrigues you as much as it does me I invite you to do your own research.

What I have proven to myself is that gratitude opens the doors wide for blessings to flow into my life; yet cultivating an attitude of gratitude costs me nothing and the rewards are limitless.

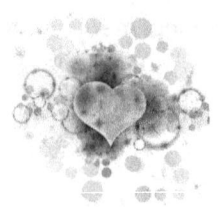

39: Affirmations and Denials

I have found affirmations to be very helpful in releasing my excess weight. You read one of my affirmations in the introduction; however, there are much simpler, easier to remember affirmations that can be used in the beginning stages of a successful weight loss program.

One of my favorites that appears to make an impact on everyone I give it to is simply:

"My world is restored to order and I am at peace."

This affirmation can be modified in numerous ways to fit your situation. I now use, "My world is in order and I am at peace" because I do not feel that any additional restoration is needed.

There are, however, things that I desire to have be true about my life that I have not yet manifested in their entirety. In that regard, I might affirm that "I am healthy, wealthy and wise."

Note that these affirmations do not include specifics. I would not affirm that "I am a tall, slender, size 8 with blue eyes." There are several reasons for not getting this specific, not the least of which are that my eyes are hazel and my body build would never realistically compact to a size 8!

The first affirmation about being healthy allows the universe to lead me to those things that will contribute to that state of health, including a weight that will be attractive for my height and frame.

Many sources of affirmations can be found on the internet by doing a search. A search for "Positive Affirmations" yielded 2,380,000 results! Though Louise Hay, the queen of positive affirmations, and one of my favorites, was on top, I chose a list from Success Consciousness: Mental Tools for a Great Life:

- I am healthy and happy.
- Wealth is pouring into my life.
- I am sailing on the river of wealth.
- I am getting wealthier each day.

Sharon Kay, M.A., L.U.T.

- My body is healthy and functioning in a very good way.
- I have a lot of energy.
- I study and comprehend fast.
- My mind is calm.
- I am calm and relaxed in every situation.
- My thoughts are under my control.
- I radiate love and happiness.
- I am surrounded by love.
- I have the perfect job for me.
- I am living in the house of my dreams.
- I have good and loving relations with my wife/husband.
- I have a wonderful and satisfying job.
- I have the means to travel abroad, whenever I want to.
- I am successful in whatever I do.
- Everything is getting better every day.

If you were to concentrate on just this list of affirmations you would cover nearly everything a person needs to lose weight and live a happy, successful life.

Another aspect that needs to be dealt with, though, is removing from our lives things (and people) that are not in alignment with our desire to lose weight and be the best person we are capable of being. This is where denials come in.

While affirmations will immediately go to work attracting good into our lives we need to release negative energy in order to make space for our good.

Linda Martella-Whitsett, in her book *How to Pray Without Talking to God*, p. 75 (2011), says that,

"I like to think of denial as spiritual Ex-Lax. In the human body, if waste cannot move through, toxicity sets in. The body is designed for release, but a buildup of stress and poor eating habits leads to constipation. Relief from acute constipation is often found in medicine that prompts elimination..

"Understanding the spiritual power of denial is like having a ready-made laxative for cases of spiritual constipation."

We may use a denial such as, "My family history of obesity has no control over me." This releases negative emotions on both a conscious and subconscious level and allows us to move forward, exercising our freedom to choose a more healthy lifestyle than our parents had taught us.

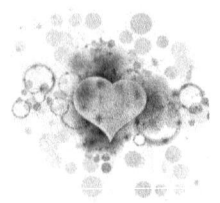

40: Finding Your Own Spiritual Path

When I found Unity Church of Christianity I learned about taking personal responsibility for my life. Overeaters Anonymous teaches much the same thing which is not surprising as the founders, Bill Wilson and Dr. Bob Smith (commonly known as Bill W. and Dr. Bob), drew heavily on the New Thought spiritual movement, of which Unity is a part. When I visited my first OA meeting in Missouri I felt the same sense of love and acceptance that I had felt with my first visit to a Unity church.

While turning our lives over to a higher power, we at the same time understand that our higher power is not forcing the fork or spoon to our mouth. I, and only I, am responsible for any aspect of my body that I have obvious control over.

For example, I was talking with a man who abuses alcohol and probably drugs. He stated to me that he didn't need to worry about whether or not he was going to heaven. His mother had told him that he was baptized and saved as an infant and was divinely protected. That, in his mind, gave him a "get out of hell free card" after death. Most people I have known who have that attitude actually long for death as an escape from their pain—yet, at the same time, live in fear of death as an unknown.

I can't disagree in that I no longer believe in hell or heaven in the afterlife. So I do not envision that man, or anyone else, going to hell when they dies. I do, however, see him creating a hell here on earth for himself and those who love him.

I can see, too, how my overeating created a hell here on earth for some of my family members. For that I am deeply regretful and I recently apologized to my son before he had the gastric bypass surgery. He forgave me a long time ago and I have forgiven myself. This is critical in the process of recovery and moving on with our lives.

Sharon Kay, M.A., L.U.T.

At the beginning of the movie "The Celestine Prophecy", based on book by the same name (1993) by James Redfield, the main character, John Woodson, is talking to a friend, Charlene. He asks her why she called him. Her reply was that, "Every time I think of this prophecy I think of you. Then I found out I had a stopover here. Maybe you are hearing this at the right time."

Throughout the movie this is a theme. I believe that whenever anyone pops into our minds there is a reason for it, rather than it being just a random thought. All of the overweight people of the world pop into my mind frequently.

I have come to treat this as a method of prayer. Whenever a name, or in this case a group of people, pop into my mind I turn it into a prayer. It can be as simple as, "Please grant them the good desires of their hearts." Or it can be whatever your higher power lays on your heart to pray.

When you pray like this, as opposed to formal prayer times, you are learning to go with the flow of the universe. You are learning to listen to your heart and this will translate into taking care of your body. This is not to say you should give up your formal times of prayer if you have a prayer practice. It is merely giving another option to those of you who believe that prayer is only effective if you set aside a specific amount of time or a set time.

Charles Fillmore, in his book *Talks on Truth* (p. 11), tells us that "It is not necessary to go in state [be formal in talking] to God. If you had a friend at your elbow at all times who could answer your every question and who loved to serve you, you certainly would not feel it necessary to go down on your knees to him or ask a favor with fear and trembling."

If you have a need and desire to lose weight my prayer is for you to find your answers on all levels—physical, mental, emotional and spiritual. You are worthy and deserving of being the best person you are capable of being. I am honored to be a part of motivating you to become that person.

Advent Sunday (November 29, 2016

Rev. Kelly Isola, in her blog "The Advent of Advent" (November 2015), tells us that **"THE SEASON of Advent is about something unknown emerging on the horizon, something we have never seen before. The word "advent" comes from the Latin adventus – to come. There is wondrous and expectant feeling about the very word 'Advent.'"** (www.kellyisola.com/the-advent-of-advent/)

Rev. Isola goes on to say that "**Advent is a quiet, contemplative time in the darkness waiting for the light, the light for the whole human race. It is a time to dig deeply into ourselves, excavating our souls, stretching our roots down to who and what we were created to be, so that we might be born anew. This inner preparation is nourished by prayer, the silence, sacred music and rituals of the season.**"

I found myself doing just that during the weekend after Thanksgiving. The weather was cold and rain misted constantly—good days to stay in a toasty warm dwelling and contemplate. And I had the freedom to do so.

I realized that I had been very, very tired from energy expended in coordinating a gala event for my church (which by all accounts was very successful). Now it was time for some "me" time.

Over the last several months I had found it very difficult to record what I ate or to record my weight on the scales. Imagine my joy at finding that I had gained only three pounds. To further compound that joy I felt ready to put as much energy into finalizing his book as I had put into the gala.

I had originally envisioned a date of January 22 for a book launch party. In the program for the gala I had a 1/2 page ad which said "Spring 2016." Honey, January in Missouri is *not* spring!

Thus I elected to delay until April 15, a Friday, tax deadline day in the U.S., should be an easy date to remember!

In the meantime ... I have some work to do. One of my favorite photographer friends took lots of photographs at the gala and at a subsequent event and I don't like the way I look even though I am happy with the way I feel.

At my best I doubt that I will ever be photogenic in front of a camera. I can, however, be at my optimal weight. See you there.

Sharon Kay, M.A., L.U.T.

After reading this section I want to _____

_____

_____

_____

_____

_____

_____

_____

_____

_____

_____

_____

_____

_____

_____

_____

_____

_____

_____

_____

_____

_____

_____

_____

PART SIX

What Are Your Environmental Issues?

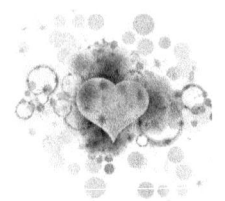

41: Preparing Your Environment

"Everything's Gonna Be Plastic By-and-By", a short-lived song of the 80s by Shel Silverstein and The Serendipity Singers made a tremendous impression on me. Today I realize that they were probably referring to credit cards, but I thought it was about Tupperware, plastic baby bottles, disposable diapers, etc., and I rebelled. "Not in my house its not." We might drink out of jelly glasses ... but they would be glass—not plastic!

At the time I first heard that song "ecology" was not a word in most people's vocabulary. I was a baby boomer and we were supposed to have the latest in technology and the easiest to take care of. The more disposable it was, the better.

I wasn't in a marriage with a lot of disposable income, however, and we had two babies. Cloth diapers, while more work, were less expensive. Glass baby bottles could be sterilized more easily—and didn't hold an odor from formula or milk. Plates that could be washed and used time after time were more frugal than paper plates. I recycled and repurposed many, many items before these became socially acceptable buzzwords.

But most important ... glass (china and crystal today) just made me feel good about myself and my family. They said, "I love you. You are important to me." Today it is critical for me to validate that for myself and they're words you need to say to yourself, *and mean them*, as you shapeshift. China and crystal may not be important to you, but the emotion of feeling good about yourself creates the impetus to move forward with being the best you can be.

A man came through our break room at work today and said, "You always have the best looking meals." My food wasn't even on good china, but it was colorful and attractively presented on a plate. Setting a mood for yourself is just as important as a romantic dinner.

Eye appeal not only appeals to the visual senses, but also gives you a feeling of satiety sooner if you enjoy the meal by eating slowly (no, you don't have to chew mashed potatoes 50 times). I hear you saying, "But I don't have time to eat slowly."

My lunch break is 30 minutes. I go to the break room, put my meal on a plate, put it in the microwave for two minutes (I like my food room temperature instead of so hot I can't taste it) and put a napkin with utensils and cooking spray on a table; then go for a comfort break. When I get back the meal is ready to put on the table and takes me about 20 minutes to actually eat—slowly.

This chapter is all about releasing anything in your environment that holds you back from being the healthiest, most attractive, loving and energetic "you" that you are capable of being. Get out your best china, crystal, flatware and cloth napkins. Stop saving them for special occasions. It is time for you to learn to love yourself and treat yourself like the queen/king that you were born to be.

Why? Psychologically we not only feel better when we treat ourselves well, but studies have shown that people eat less when food is presented attractively and colorfully. Forget about paper plates ... or, worse yet, eating out of the can over the sink. (Look me in the eyes and tell me you've never done that.)

I cannot intuit what in your environment needs to be changed in order to facilitate your weight loss, but areas that I had to change include:

Reorganizing my kitchen—I cannot count the number of times I've thrown away or, a little better, given away lots of good food—that wasn't good for me. It is okay, though. I'm sure you've heard the saying, "Better to go to waste than to go to waist."

Turning off the TV—In 2010, after divorcing, I bought a nice big television—which I have never used as a TV. I get DVDs from the public library, occasionally buying one that is so good that I want to share it with friends, and selectively watch what I want to view.

It is better now that there are ways to choose not to view commercials, but even sitcoms bombard you with scenes of people cooking, drinking wine, etc.—and, of course, none of them need to lose an ounce!

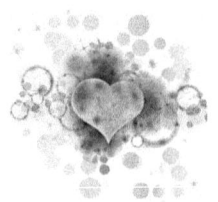

42: Dress for Success

Camouflage is key to taking pounds off your appearance. You've probably heard that the camera puts 10-pounds on in photographs. After the photo shoot for the covers of this book I can attest to that fact! Dressing properly can take 10-pounds off.

Standing up straight as I learned to do with the help of a chiropractor can also make a huge difference in your appearance. His suggestions and my work quickly taught me that targeted exercises could noticeably reduce the appearance of my having an abnormally large posterior. This overcame a major obstacle to my feeling good about my appearance. An important note—these were exercises that I could do sitting in a chair!

Now, even though I feel better about my butt, I focus on highlighting my positives and taking a person's attention off the area below my waist. I do this by wearing solid color slimming slacks or skirt with a vibrant, low cut blouse, with or without flowing jacket.

When you get serious about losing weight you are going to need new clothes soon. If you need to lose as much as I needed to lose it doesn't make sense to buy new clothes, not even from low cost outlet stores.

It is amazing, however, how many beautiful, fashionable clothes, often with tags still on them, you can find at your local Goodwill, Salvation Army, or other thrift stores and garage sales. My workplace has an area where employees can leave good condition clothes that they no longer want and take anything they like. Try it—you'll like the sense of saving money and helping someone else dress for success at the same time.

Last week my boss walked in—wearing one of my outfits! Well, not mine, but identical to mine. When I commented on this, she told me where she had bought it. I said, "I found mine at a thrift shop."

"Even better," she proclaimed with a smile. Thankfully, buying smart is no longer frowned upon by intelligent women as it once was.

I learned the secret, and I'm proud of it, when my children were little. When money is tight it does not make sense to spend $50-$100 on a new dress for a five-year-old girl who will likely get chocolate on it the first time she wears it. Translate that into buying clothes for mom, as well.

After losing weight the first time, I went to a church garage sale, told the women holding the sale about the weight I had lost and that if they would bring me everything they had in a specific size that I would buy everything that fit and looked good on me. They did and I did.

I walked out of there feeling like royalty for less than $20. Clothes do not have to be new to be new to you. In most of today's society, fashion is what you make it. Thank God, it is no longer a mortal sin to combine black with brown (as it was in my Mother's day) or to wear white shoes in winter months.

Whatever you do, though, get rid of clothes that no longer fit. Sloppy is *not* in! I went through my closet with an eye for things that no longer fit or were not flattering on me and released them.

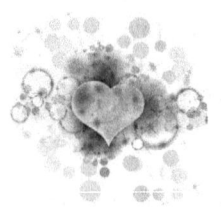

43: Toxic Environments

Last night during a meeting a friend brought up the subject of how plants know what nutrients to absorb from the soil they're planted in. As a person with a curious journalist's mindset, I went home and did an internet search.

Wikipedia, in an article on plant nutrition, says that, "E. Epstein defined two criteria for an element to be essential for plant growth: 1) in its absence the plant is unable to complete a normal life cycle; or 2) that the element is part of some essential plant constituent or metabolite."

How do plants know what nutrients to absorb from the soil? They don't. They simply draw whatever is available. As a result, some thrive, some die, and there are many stages of health or disease in between.

It occurred to me that we, as humans, are not so much different. I am currently in an environment that is rich in nutrients that allow me to thrive and prosper.

A new colleague at work has commented "you are so sweet" because I give out hugs and smiles liberally. I'm only able to do so because of my environment. I absorb positive energy everywhere I go—work, church, social groups, even my apartment complex.

It hasn't always been like that. My second husband frequently said that he was attracted to me because of my smiles. Yet he did nothing to keep that smile on my face and did his best to isolate me from friends and family.

What about you? Are you in an environment where you can thrive, grow, flourish? If not, do you have the power to make changes? The answer is, "Yes!" However, making changes may mean sacrificing more than we are willing to sacrifice.

Do you find yourself complaining frequently to friends or other family members about your situation? Then do something about it. This is rather indelicate, but my mother used to tell me, "S*** or get off the pot!" Do something, even if it is wrong. Add spice to the mix. Remove something, or someone, from the mix.

Sharon Kay, M.A., L.U.T.

If you are in a relationship that is toxic to you, there is no way that you are going to lose weight. That toxicity undermines any chance you have to lose weight. You are going to have to decide whether the relationship is worth the price that you are paying in order to maintain a semblance of what you consider a normal lifestyle.

In my work as director of a crisis center for abused women and children I met wealthy women who put up with black eyes and broken arms because leaving the abusive relationship would mean leaving not only their social status, but possibly their children. A court usually awards custody to the partner with money to support the children in the lifestyle to which they were accustomed.

In most of these circumstances the women have been stay-at-home-moms, with no jobs and no personal bank accounts, who could not provide the things that our society considers important.

But being miserable and suffering, is not normal either.

There are two terms that I find useful in defining unhealthy environments—one that you allow and one that you create:

Psychic Vampires—No, I'm not going occultish on you. I'm not talking about creatures that come out only at night and suck blood. I am talking about times when you find yourself around someone, or doing something, that drains your energy. You feel a need to escape.

The person may or may not be aware of their effect on you. In either case, you are the only one who can decide whether or not the relationship is worth the investment you are making in it. Understand, though, that you are "spending" energy on that person and if they are not capable of returning the energy you will feel depleted.

Energy Leaks—These are ways you spend energy needlessly and you create the leaks yourself. The best illustration I have heard is of having a lightbulb that needs to be changed. Every time you walk by the lamp or fixture you think, "I have to get around to replacing that bulb." Then you walk off.

The next day ... and the next ... and the next ... same thing.

These are all needless energy expenditures that are not necessary. Buy a package of four bulbs and keep them on hand. You'll need them sometime in the future. The first time you notice that a bulb is out take two minutes to replace it; then you won't have to waste energy thinking about it.

> WHEN PEOPLE UNDERMINE YOUR DREAMS,
> PREDICT YOUR DOOM OR CRITICIZE YOU,
> REMEMBER THEY'RE TELLING YOU THEIR STORY,
> NOT YOURS.

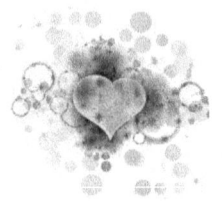

44: Tools of the Trade - For the Kitchen

The following are items that I consider "must haves" in order to keep track of what you are actually putting in your mouth or to make it easy to take foods you can eat to work.

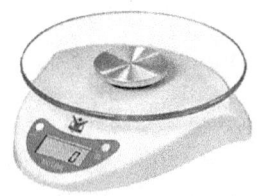

Kitchen Scales (ounces and grams)— These do not need to be the expensive scales that will calculate everything for you, save records of items you eat frequently, etc. I like "bells and whistles" on my cell phone, but they are entirely unnecessary on kitchen scales. I bought my Taylor brand at Bed, Bath & Beyond for $19.99. This is funny, though. Remember my criticism of "The World's Biggest Loser"? I noticed when I went to the kitchen to check my brand that it has a small "The Biggest Loser" logo! I probably would not buy that brand again because of my opinion of that show, though the scale has given excellent service. The same store also has a Salter brand for the same price which appears comparable.

Measuring Cups and spoons—I use measuring cups for many items, though you could actually weigh them by the ounce or gram. You can buy a good set of plastic cups or spoons for $1.00 at a local Dollar Tree or comparable store in your area, if you don't already have sets, and I find them good to have around.

Glass Bowls—I find it to be incredibly useful in planning my meals to have see-through bowls of fruits, vegetables and main dishes which are pre-measured. All I have to do is take 3-4 out of the refrigerator, put them in my lunch box and I'm ready to go. Bowls pictured were found at Crate & Barrel for $19.95 per dozen.

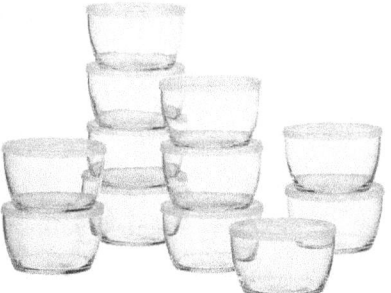

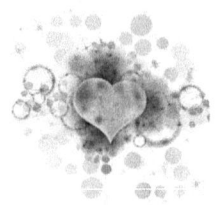

45: Tools of the Trade - For the Pantry

Vegetables—A friend of mine has a severe aversion to vegetables, especially green ones, which are the lowest calorie, lowest Weight Watchers point count. It seems strange to me because I love cooked broccoli, asparagus, brussels sprouts, etc. Other people, however, consider them only a step above eating grass!

My mother-in-law, the one who taught me how to cook country style, had a similar challenge. When she developed heart trouble the doctor told her to lose weight and concentrate on vegetables. The problem was that vegetables to her were corn and potatoes—even macaroni and cheese because it is a side dish!

There is nothing wrong with corn and potatoes and, in fact, I eat a lot of them. But I use them as a bread substitute instead of vegetables. As bread substitutes they are excellent choices over breads which, even with the highest fiber enriched types, have additives and preservatives. They're also good for you as vegetable nutrition, too. Just remember that:

1 Potato medium (2-1/4" to 3-1/4" dia) = 163 calories/4 points
2/3 cup corn kernels = 70 calories/2 points
10 asparagus spears = 30 calories/0 points
1 cup summer squash, sliced = 18 calories/0 points
1 cup broccoli, chopped = 50 calories/0 points

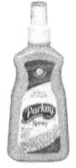 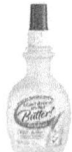 **0-Calorie Butter Flavored Spray**—Spray any of the vegetables above, after cooking with I Can't Believe It's Not Butter or Parkay 0-calorie butter flavored sprays, sprinkle with salt and pepper and enjoy. They are delicious! I simply microwave slices or chunks of many vegetables in a microwavable plastic bag until they are the tenderness I prefer.

Sharon Kay, M.A., L.U.T.

Use this type spray as a substitute anywhere you would ordinarily use melted butter or margarine. Yes, olive oil may be healthier, but when we're eating to lose weight, calories count. One tablespoon of olive oil has 120 calories. Use it sparingly.

Coffee—While we're comparing, let's compare coffee and additions to coffee. I drink quite a bit of coffee and experience no adverse side effects though, admittedly, that may be because I don't drink it very strong. You've read elsewhere that I have one really rich cup of coffee at night with cookies as an end-of-the-day dessert treat.

During the day, however, I drink flavored coffees black. Right now my favorites are "Ripe Red Cherry" and "Blueberry Crumble" flavors. They don't have enough calories per cup to make it necessary to count and I enjoy the flavors. If you drink coffee, consider this:

1 cup coffee, black = 0 calories/0 points

1 cup coffee, with 3 tablespoons creamer and 5 teaspoons sugar = 120 calories/3 points (I know you are looking at that "5 teaspoons sugar" with shock, but consider that one 12 ounce can of Coke contains over 9 teaspoons !

1 cup (8 ounces) Starbucks White Chocolate Mocha (my favorite) = 270 calories/7 points. But who buys an eight ounce cup? A 12 ounce cup is $3.65 compared to $4.65 for 20 ounces. Perhaps part of my weight problem has been buying the best value for my dollar!

Coconut Oil—Years ago I read that coconut oil would stimulate thyroid function and I tried it ... but not for long. The recommended consumption was three tablespoons per day and, at 120 calories per tablespoon, that didn't fit any diet I've ever been on. However, when I read the following I am convinced that coconut oil is the only oil we should have in our pantries and it is the one for me.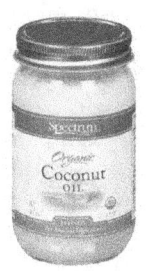

I have cited some benefits of coconut oil in an earlier chapter, but www.organidfacts.net has this to say:

"The health benefits of coconut oil include hair care, skin care, stress relief, cholesterol level maintenance, weight loss, boosted immune system, proper digestion and regulated metabolism. It also provides relief from kidney problems, heart diseases, high blood pressure, diabetes, HIV, and cancer, while helping to improve dental quality and bone strength. These benefits of oil can be attributed to the presence of lauric acid, capric acid and caprylic acid, and their respective properties, such as antimicrobial, antioxidant, anti-fungal, antibacterial and soothing qualities."

Lean Meats (protein equivalent for vegetarians and vegans)— We all need protein to build muscle and I have read that our need for protein increases as we age. I have some lean protein with nearly every meal. Rather than going vegetarian, or vegan, I choose to eat meat in moderation. Compared to huge portions of barbecued meat that my family used to eat, I am saving the lives of many animals.

A normal size serving of protein for me is 2-4 ounces and I prefer pre-packaged so that it is easy to control portion size. As I write this book, one of my favorite meals is Chicken Cordon Bleu. For those of you not familiar with this recipe, it is chicken breast pounded thin, a slice of ham and some cheese rolled inside the chicken. The meat and cheese are then rolled in bread crumbs.

I buy them pre-formed, frozen, in boxes of four. A portion is 230 calories and all the cooking that is required is unwrapping one, putting it on an ovenproof metal sheet and baking for 35 minutes. Pair that with a baked potato or potatoes au gratin (Betty Crocker mix—25 minutes) and some asparagus or broccoli for a delicious dinner.

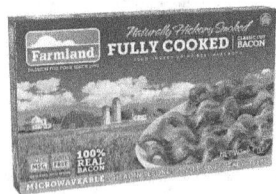 One of my favorite proteins is bacon and I still eat it. The change I have made is to use precooked bacon. I especially like it for its ease in preparation—there is no greasy cleaning up afterwards. 25 seconds in the microwave and it is ready. It tastes like the real thing because it is the real thing! The only difference is that most of the fat has been pressed out. I eat it for breakfast with gluten-free blueberry pancakes and make bacon, lettuce and tomato sandwiches occasionally. Three slices for three points is a flavorful addition to any meal .

Almond Milk—I avoid most milk and products containing milk. I tried using coconut milk as a substitute. It tastes good and, if coconut oil is good for me, the milk of a coconut should be good for me, too. Right? Wrong. After drinking my first coconut milk I got horrible gas—the same kind of gas that people who are lactose intolerant get. It did not take long for me to figure out that the only change in my diet had been the coconut milk. I changed to almond milk. Problem resolved. I am allergic to, or extremely intolerant of, coconut milk.

The only thing I have found that you cannot do with almond milk is to use it in making instant puddings. You get a milkshake!

Gluten-Free Bread—I avoid wheat as much as possible. I get my starch carbs primarily from vegetables, but there are times when a meal just needs bread to be complete. Although it has improved tremendously and is readily available in many stores, gluten-free bread slices and rolls still leave a lot to be desired in texture and taste.

Primarily I use gluten-free pancakes and waffles which I find to be perfectly acceptable substitutes for wheat-based equivalents. The ones I buy are frozen and easy to pop into a toaster or microwave for quick and easy breakfasts before going to work.

40-45-Calorie Breads—After writing the previous section I found myself craving sandwiches which is almost unheard of for me. But I bought some 40-calorie per slice Nature's Own Honey Wheat bread (1 point per slice). It is not your grandmother's low-calorie bread. It is light, tastes delicious and is very satisfying.

My favorite fillings at this moment are: 1) a 2-ounce package of Buddig ultrathin shaved meat (ham, pastrami, beef, chicken) (90-100 calories/2 points), fat-free mayonnaise, lettuce, tomato and onion; or 2) Curly's Pulled Beef with barbecue sauce (1/4 cup = 60 calories/2 points) with a big slice of sweet raw onion. Either of these is very satisfying for very few calories or points.

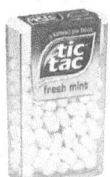

Tic-Tacs—I keep a box of Tic Tac Fresh Mints in my car and one in my purse. If I'm feeling the need to put something in my mouth I use one of them. At 2-calories per mint they leave a cool, refreshing taste and improve my breath.

Vitamins—I'm putting vitamins in here as essential because I think this is an important safeguard, but I don't go overboard. I take a store brand (bought when they are buy 1 get 1 free) multi-vitamin for women over 50. And, because my doctor prescribed it, I take 2000 IU of vitamin D. He says that very few people, especially in northern states, get enough D.

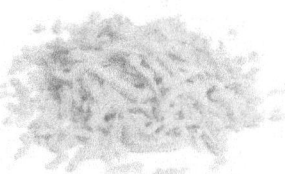

Grated Sharp Cheddar Cheese -- An ounce of shredded cheese seems like a lot more than a domino-sized rectangle of the same cheese.

Egg Substitute—Egg Beaters is probably the best known egg substitute and is the one I have shown. However, there are less expensive brands which I have used successfully. Basically, egg substitute consists of egg whites which have coloring, spices and other additives to give them the color and consistency of whole beaten eggs.

The advantage to using egg substitutes on a low calorie diet is that they average one-third the calories—or you can have three times as much. A large whole egg has 90 calories. The equivalent in Egg Beaters has 25 calories, nearly as much protein and no fat.

Fat Free Mayonnaise—The advantage to fat free mayonnaise, much like egg substitute, is lower calories. One tablespoon of Kraft fat free mayonnaise is 10 calories compared to 90 calories in the same amount of full fat.

I find the texture and flavor to be very acceptable when spread on bread for sandwiches or used in dishes like potato salad. It can also be mixed with various other sauces or spices to create flavors you like. I mix it with mustard, to taste, to spread on ham or roast beef sandwiches (maybe a little horseradish, too). Mix it with ketchup and pickles for a variation of thousand island dressing. Experiment!

Mustard—If you like mustard you get a lot of flavor for very few calories. Growing up in Texas I learned that potato salad isn't the real thing if it doesn't have mustard in it and lots of dill pickle, onion and pimiento. None of these additions have a significant number of calories and they stretch the size of a serving considerable.

Flavorful Sauces—There are numerous brands of sauces on grocery stores shelves that can add flavor to proteins and vegetables. I show Lawry's because I have their Szechuan sweet & Sour BBQ and Caribbean Jerk in my refrigerator at the present time.

I enjoy these very much and at 30-35 calories to a tablespoon of intense flavor are a good addition to your menu. Lawry's calls these "marinades," but don't think the only way to use them is to soak meat in them before cooking. I cook roast pork or chicken and simply brush 1/2 to 1 tablespoon of the sauce on the meat just before serving. It is wonderful!

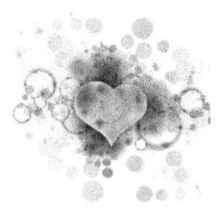

46: Release These!

Nutrition Bars—Bet you can't eat just one nutrition bar any more than you can eat just one potato chip! Therein lies the problem for me. There's really not anything wrong with a good quality bar, and there are nut and dried fruit bars that are gluten-free, but they are not low in calories as a rule and I find it very difficult to stop at just one. They're too much like eating a candy bar, have almost as many calories and aren't filling. For something to be good for me on a diet it has to meet a satiety quotient. In other words, I need to feel comfortably full after eating it.

NOTE: I may have just made an exception. Someone brought some gluten-free bars to work to give away. I took one chocolate and one caramel apple bar. The next morning I had the caramel apple bar with a glass of milk before going to work and found that it kept me satisfied for an extended period of time. I had actually taken the second bar to work, planned it into my meal allowance for the day, and found that I didn't need it. I'm having the chocolate bar tonight with my coffee for dessert.

That is one of the pluses of this type program—adjust to meet your preferences and lifestyle needs. This would be a good bar for me if I were away from home more.

Nutrition Drinks—I, personally, have not found one that I like. Spiru-Tein plant-based protein with spirulina has only 99 calories per serving (plus milk added) and was incredibly good for me while I had ulcers in my bladder and didn't know it. I could go on a diet of Spiru-Tein, even adding fruit such as a banana or apple in a blender, and my pain would go away.

One problem for me was that it turned thick, slimy—and green—very quickly and even though the taste wasn't bad I could not tolerate it for many days in a row.

Expensive Steaks—Do you know why they're expensive? They have more marbled fat content; thus, more flavor and they are more tender. It is not difficult, though, to take a less tender piece of beef, learn different ways to tenderize it and flavor with spices.

Butter and Margarine—Butter and margarine, from what I read, have very little other than flavor to contribute to a balanced diet. They are definitely "red light" foods for me. One of my guilty little secrets ... if my mind is on a bender/binge, I can eat real, salted butter straight out of the package sans bread! It is not worth it to me.

I now have only coconut oil in the house for cooking which I use 1/2 teaspoon (20 calories) at a time when I want to brown potato slices or maybe stir-fry.

For the flavor of butter for vegetables I use Parkay's 0-calorie spray which is cholesterol and trans fat-free. A spritz is 0 calories, but you can pretty much spray all you want and not do any damage to a diet. I don't count it and I carry a bottle in my lunch box every day. I Can't Believe It's Not Butter brand has the same type spray, but where I live I find it to be much more expensive than Parkay.

Most Canned Vegetables—In general, nutrients in vegetables go from high in frozen to medium in fresh and low in canned. In addition to being low in nutrients, canned vegetables usually contain a lot of salt as a flavor enhancer and preservative. Canned tomatoes are, however, actually one fruit (not a vegetable) whose nutrient value increases when canned.

According to Gene Lester, Ph.D., a research plant physiologist at the USDA's Food Quality Lab in Beltsville, MD, that's because canning calls for heating, which causes certain raw vegetables, such as corn and tomatoes, to release antioxidants and make them more nutritionally available. (www.eatingwell.com)

But why, you ask, frozen as opposed to fresh?

Do you have any idea how long "fresh" fruits and vegetables have been sitting somewhere before going on your grocer's shelf for sale? Tomatoes that are picked green and gassed to ripen are just one example. Vegetables fresh from your garden or a friend's are wonderful, but many of us do not have easy access to REALLY fresh produce.

Sharon Kay, M.A., L.U.T.

Most Chips—The only chips I usually have in my home are tortilla chips. Most of the time I can handle a one-ounce weighed serving which I will top with one-ounce of cheddar cheese and some pickled jalapeno slices for nachos. Or I make my own homemade bean dip from canned fat-free refried beans (recipe page __) and eat some with a serving of chips. It is hard to go overboard very much with bean dip.

Most Cookies and Candy—Cookies and candy are dangerous foods for my diet, but I find that I can keep lemon and ginger thins on hand and portion-control them easily. One cookie is about 20 calories. They are light, crisp, high in flavor and very satisfying.

Alcoholic Beverages—This is easy for me to say because I've never been a fan of any alcoholic beverages except for mixed drinks like Margaritas that are really nothing but high octane sugar syrup! The problem with any alcoholic beverage or sugar-laden soft drink is that it is possible to consume hundreds of calories without realizing what you are doing.

Soft Drinks—See above, with the exception of sugar-free. I know that there are many studies about the health risks of sweeteners like Aspartame, but we have to make informed choices and I choose to drink sugar-free soft drinks in moderation. My favorite at the present time is A&W Diet Root Beer. To me, and I have heard others say the same, it is like a liquid dessert with rich taste and no after-taste. I buy them by the 2-litre bottle and drink about one bottle a week as an after work refresher. For me this is much better than an after work beer or cocktail.

Vending Machines at Work—Though, technically, you probably don't have the authority to actually get rid of vending machines where you work, you do have the choice of whether to pay for high priced items in them. I went through a period of buying a Payday candy bar every afternoon out of our machine—and getting upset when the machine had run out of them! I needed the "nutrition" of that bar's 240 calories as much as I needed an extra hole in my head. But they are gluten-free!

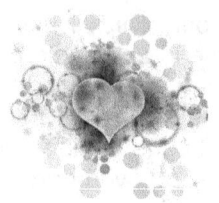

47: Reading Labels

I love grocery shopping and reading labels. I love trying new foods ... experimenting with tastes and textures. Not all food items, however, fit easily into a weight reduction program and that is where reading labels becomes important.

When my children were young and there were four mouths to feed I used a lot of coupons. At that time, in Texas, stores would double and often triple the face value—often resulting in free items. I could always find a way to incorporate low and no-cost food items into our diet, but they weren't always the healthiest choices.

Today, cooking for only myself and more conscious of what I put into my body, reading labels is more important.

For example, I made sausage jambalaya with okra pods for dinner this evening. I choose Hillshire Farms smoked turkey sausage links for this dish. Why? Consider the labels on the opposite page.

The label on the left. Is the one that I used. Two ounces has 90 calories, 5 grams fat, 8 grams protein and 2 carbohydrates which equals 2 points on my plan.

Now look at the label on the right. It is from the same Hillshire Farms family, but there are some major differences. This one is their beef sausage which has 190 calories for the same two ounces, 17 grams fat, 7 grams protein and 1 carbohydrate. The point count for this option is 5 points - two and one-half times as many.

In my opinion, the turkey sausage is just as flavorful and enjoyable as the beef and saves me a lot of calories and points.

For those of you who watch your salt you will notice that there is slightly more sodium in the turkey sausage, but the difference is not significant.

Sharon Kay, M.A., L.U.T.

Nutrition Facts

Serving Size: 2 oz (56g)

Amount Per Serving	
Calories 90	Calories from Fat 45

	% Daily Value*
Total Fat 5 g	8%
Saturated Fat 2 g	10%
Trans Fat 0 g	
Cholesterol 35 mg	12%
Sodium 510 mg	21%
Potassium	
Total Carbohydrate 2 g	1%
Dietary Fiber 0 g	0%
Sugars 2 g	
Sugar Alcohols 0 g	
Protein 8 g	
Vitamin A 0 IU	0%
Vitamin C 1.2 mg	2%
Calcium 0 mg	0%
Iron 0.36 mg	2%

Nutrition Facts

Serving Size: 2 oz (56g)

Amount Per Serving	
Calories 190	Calories from Fat 150

	% Daily Value*
Total Fat 17 g	26%
Saturated Fat 8 g	40%
Trans Fat 1 g	
Cholesterol 40 mg	13%
Sodium 460 mg	19%
Potassium	
Total Carbohydrate 1 g	0%
Dietary Fiber 0 g	0%
Sugars 1 g	
Sugar Alcohols 0 g	
Protein 7 g	
Vitamin A 0 IU	0%
Vitamin C 1.2 mg	2%
Calcium 0 mg	0%
Iron 0.72 mg	4%

Many more comparisons could be made, but the important thing is for you to learn to read labels yourself. It is also important to use your judgment as to their accuracy.

I found a brand of pancake syrup that says there are 100 calories in 1/4 cup. Considering that most pancake syrup says 200 calories per 1/4 cup, I questioned the accuracy to the point that I contacted the company which did not give me a satisfactory answer. They have a lite version, but the bottle I have (rechecked accuracy after writing this) does not say "lite."

By that time I had decided that I prefer one tablespoon of real maple syrup to pancake syrup, but it is important to question if something on a label does not sound realistic and you really want to eat that brand.

Portion Control

Another reason for learning to read labels is to learn how much the company considers a "serving" to be. What looks like a moderate amount to you and me may actually be 2-3 servings, in which case the calorie count increases dramatically.

For example, if you drink a 20 ounce bottle of sugar (or high fructose corn syrup) sweetened Coke you are consuming 100 calories, right?

Current Label	Proposed Label

Nutrition Facts

Serving Size 8 fl oz (240 mL)
Servings Per Container about 2.5

Amount Per Serving	
Calories 110	
	% Daily Value*
Total Fat 0g	0%
Sodium 70mg	3%
Total Carbohydrate 31g	10%
Sugars 30g	
Protein 0g	

*Percent Daily Values are based on a 2,000 calorie diet

Nutrition Facts

Serving Size 1 bottle (600 mL)
Servings Per Container 1

Amount Per Serving	% Daily Value*
Calories 275	14%
Total Fat 0g	0%
Sodium 175mg	7%
Total Carbohydrate 78g	26%
Sugars 75g	
Protein 0g	

*Percent Daily Values are based on a 2,000 calorie diet

Wrong.

Under current labeling guidelines a 20 ounce bottle of Coke is 2 1/2 servings of 110 each for a total of 275 calories.

Be prepared for many shocks when you began paying attention to labels. Though the United States has many labeling laws, and the label above is accurate, it is also misleading if you don't understand what information to look for.

Sharon Kay, M.A., L.U.T.

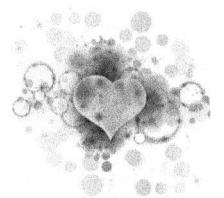

48: Financing This Venture

By the time you are reading this chapter you may be wondering why the meals that I ate were so low cost. Obviously this book has done well, I continued to work full time while writing the book, and I had social security income. So why did I choose to eat meals that some people would consider near poverty level?

Why, too, did I choose to eat processed foods that my natural, organic, fresh foods friends would consider low nutrition?

I ate the way I did in order to show that it is possible to lose weight on a low budget and not feel deprived.

Yes, I did eat nicer meals out with my friends, but I did those as a form of entertainment which I consider to be necessary for the normal, healthy individual. We are not, "islands unto ourselves," but social individuals who do much better when in the company of people with similar interests.

My friends understand my need to watch my calorie intake and are always amenable to going to any restaurant I choose. In that way I enjoy their company and have the option of staying on my weight loss program. Do I always? You know I don't. I am just as human as you are and just as fallible. The difference is that after I have gone off program I get right back on—and I don't Sharon bash!

If you are still buying chips, candy bars, huge steaks, donuts and other rich desserts, ice cream, etc., I will wager that you are spending more money on groceries per person than I spend. "Staying on a diet costs more than I spend on groceries!" you say. Wrong.

My dinner as I write this tonight consists of a lean pork loin slice ($1.00), 1/3-pound fresh asparagus (33-cents) and a 5 1/2 ounce baked potato (10-cents). After dinner I will have a cup of coffee (10-cents), with 5 teaspoons raw sugar (10-cents) and 3 tablespoons liquid coffee creamer (7-cents); plus 8 lemon thin cookies (42-cents). The total for this meal is $2.12. How much did you spend on that Kentucky Fried Chicken dinner?

What you are asking is, "How did you buy asparagus for 99-cents a pound?" I comparison shop and eat vegetables that are in season. Asparagus is one of my favorites and at this price I'll eat it several times this week.

Recently a friend talked about how proud she was for avoiding the vending machines at her workplace. I know those machines, loaded with chips, candy bars, and other high calorie snack items, costing from $0.60 to a $1.25, and I'm proud of her, too.

I didn't say anything, but I wonder if she's putting the money saved into a fund for rewarding herself. It may not seem like much each time you put the money into a vending machine, but dollars add up fast.

Think how much you would save in a month, for example, if you are a person who stops at Starbucks on the way to work every morning for a $5 latte! It wouldn't take long to have a new designer dress hanging in your closet.

As you lose weight, go through your closet and, as my friend told me, get rid of everything that doesn't make heads turn when you walk in the door. If you haven't worn it in six months you probably aren't going to wear it. A spiritual law is that you have to get rid of things before new can flow in.

As I buy something that is new to me, I find something in the closet that I don't wear for some reason. Either it doesn't fit me the way I would like it to fit or I just don't like it any longer. So I donate it to an organization that will see to it that someone will get it who will love and appreciate it.

If you are fortunate to have friends whose sizes fluctuate start a swap pantry. We have a giveaway section at work and I picked up many nice items while losing weight.

Where there's a will, there's a way. Losing weight does not have to break your family's bank account.

I would bet that by the time you've lost 40-pounds you will either receive a promotion on your job or have changed to a better paying job because you now have the motivation, confidence and stamina to excel at what you do.

Sharon Kay, M.A., L.U.T.

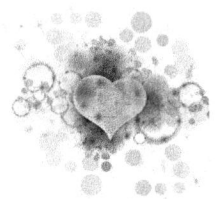

49: Less is More

When I divorced my second husband, one of the things I asked for was the cookbooks. I was thinking about ones I had bought. What he sent me was ALL the cookbooks in the house which included many expensive collectible cookbooks from the last several decades! For example, Julia Child's *Mastering the Art of French Cooking* and *The French Chef* with recipes calling for cream, butter and lots of sugar.

I remember that one of my favorite statements in my years of rearing a family, and after the children were grown, was that having a freezer full of food was more security than money in the bank for me.

It has taken years to release that obsession. Gradually, often against my will and not all that long ago as of this 2015 writing, I was forced to give up quantities. Today I buy only enough for 2-3 days rather than hoarding or stockpiling foodstuff. It may have been okay to purchase quantities of items on sale when I was feeding a family of four, but I can no longer rationalize that behavior as "saving money by buying on sale."

Today I still watch for sales, but buy only what I can use within a reasonable amount of time. Having excess food around that I can easily prepare (or eat straight out of the bag, cabinet or freezer) is a recipe for a binge. It is far better for me to buy just the amount I need for a week of lunches and dinners than to "stock up" on sales.

Frozen vegetables are an exception. When one-pound bags of peas, corn, mixed vegetables and green beans are on sale for less than $1.00 a bag I stock up. I will cook one, or sometimes two, bags at a time and portion them out into glass containers for "grab-and-go" lunch additions.

In the case of peas and corn, they can be portioned straight out of the bag frozen and quick cooked in the microwave when I'm ready to eat lunch. At the table I spritz with butter-flavored spray and sprinkle with salt and pepper, as desired.

If I were to compulsively overeat any of the cooked vegetables, including starchy corn and peas, it probably would not have any effect on the scales due to their fiber content. Unfortunately, how many people have you ever heard say, "I just can't get enough broccoli!"

In fact, a tip I learned from Weight Watchers is to cook a big pot of soup using only low-calorie (0-point) vegetables and keep it in the refrigerator. Use it for a snack when you feel hungry before a meal or for a midnight raid on the refrigerator. Use a lot of your favorite spices and it is very satisfying.

One key to "less is more" is to know what is in your pantry. Yesterday I bought three kinds of meat. I knew that I had fresh zucchini, broccoli and green beans already cooked and potatoes and rice mixes on hand. All I needed to go with them for next week was sources of protein which, for me, is usually meat.

Identify what are called "red light" foods—things that once you get started eating them you have trouble stopping such as potato chips,

Disclaimer: Many French people are not as heavy as many Americans in spite of apparent dietary overload, but what we don't see is that they eat tiny portions of rich food, savoring every bite as perfection, as opposed to gorging like we do—and they walk a lot.

candy, etc. I find that I can handle one box at a time of cookie thins (British style crisp cookies with 20 calories per cookie), portioning them out with my coffee at night, but if I bought soft white chocolate and macadamia nut cookies (you know the kind I'm talking about) I could still eat a box full in one sitting.

The idea of buying after a holiday 90% off candy, cookies, etc., is strictly taboo. And those baskets as you come in the door of a grocery store after Halloween or Christmas can be very tempting. This is the time to have blinders on. Ten-cent bags of chocolates are not a bargain!

Another good example of keeping it simple is coffee. In spite of the fact that I have a rich cup of coffee at night, the rest of the day I drink my coffee black. As mentioned previously, I like flavored coffee. I buy 1.75-ounce bags at WalMart and one bag makes 10 cups of reasonably strong coffee for me. At $1.00 per bag, that's 10-cents per cup using reusable Keurig filters at work.

I can remember spending many of my waking hours thinking about what I would cook for the next meal, scouring magazines and cookbooks for interesting new recipes, shopping for ingredients, meal preparation, having friends over to show off my latest creations ... my world revolved around food.

I thought I was just doing what good wives and mothers do, but in hindsight I can see how my need to be around food actually translated into compulsive behavior. If I wasn't cooking or eating I was thinking about what I would cook or eat. Today I have so many other more interesting things to think about. Meals come together quickly and easily as I identify meats and prepackaged frozen main dish items that are quick and easy to prepare.

Less is more, too, when consider vegetable choices. When I talk about potatoes I am talking about fresh potatoes with added low-calorie flavorings, not mashed potatoes loaded with butter and cream or scalloped potatoes loaded with butter, cheese and cream. And corn is fresh corn-on-the-cob or frozen corn kernels. If you think canned cream style corn is corn—read the label! In addition to corn it includes cornstarch and sugar, the latter being the reason it tastes so delightfully sweet.

Earlier I mentioned my former husband handing me a list of foods he liked. Today I could make a similar list. Mine would be expanded, but my requirements for a nutritious, varied diet take little time and energy to prepare. That leaves me needing less time to grocery shop and prepare meals and more time to go to social activities. Yours will be different than mine, but I have a variety of groups I attend nearly every evening of the week.

Perhaps you like to go bowling or fishing - just skip the snacks and enjoy the atmosphere and company.

- - - - -

There is one area where more is helpful—spices/flavorings. I choose sharp cheddar instead of mild because it takes less to satisfy the taste buds. Full fat dressings and marinades for the same reason.

When I was young I wanted french fries with my catsup instead of catsup with my french fries—flavor. Although I now love a plain baked potato with a spritz of buttery spray and salt, it can seem rather dry and lifeless if you are not accustomed to the taste without it dripping in butter, sour cream and cheese. Try dipping it in catsup!

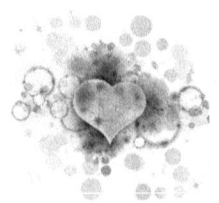

50: Dress Up a TV dinner

Before divorcing, my husband and I began a restoration of our home. For months I was without a kitchen and most meals were cooked in a microwave. Frustration after frustration had me eating less than nutritious meals, including baked goods that were loaded with fat and sugar—and calories. This, of course, led to a gain of several pounds and, after working so hard to lose over 100-pounds in 1995/96, I could not allow myself to continue desecrating my body temple.

A careful analysis over a Christmas holiday revealed to me that I was eating lots of TV dinners. And, unlike my experiences with TV dinners when my children were young (when I swore that they weren't fit for swine), today's TV dinners can actually be quite tasty, low in fat, calories and sodium if you choose the right ones, and some are reasonably nutritious.

The key to enjoying TV dinners is to dress them up. I buy Lean Cuisine, Healthy Choice or Weight Watchers brands (whichever is on sale) which contain a protein and a starch, but not a vegetable. Before you cook the dinner microwave a package of non-starch vegetables such as a broccoli and cauliflower mix, oriental mix, asparagus mix or green beans until tender (usually 5-6 minutes). Set them aside. Cook the TV dinner following instructions on the box.

While the vegetables and TV dinner are cooking set a nice table with your best china, silverware, crystal and napkin with napkin holder. Put a slice of light multi-grain bread or roll on a bread plate with a teaspoon of organic coconut oil. Pour yourself a glass of tea or ice water or a diet Coke. Arrange the contents of the TV dinner and a cup or more of vegetables on the plate. Spray vegetables with 0 calorie spray and salt (if you are not on a sodium restricted diet).

Turn the TV off, relax and enjoy every savory mouthful. Even better ... invite a friend or two over and multiply the enjoyment with good conversation.

Sharon Kay, M.A., L.U.T.

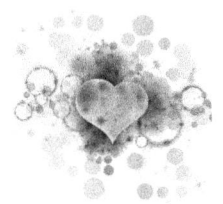

51: Dining Out

Growing up with a mother who was a school teacher, tired each evening after dealing with issues involving students and parents, and remember that she hated to cook, we ate out every night. Though I learned to cook, and loved doing so, dining out was a hard habit to break when I got married.

In retrospect (doesn't everything seem so much simpler when we can look back with more mature understanding), my husband and I would have had "date nights" to satisfy my need while enjoying my home cooking the rest of the week.

Today I still enjoy eating out and do so frequently. The differences are that I:

1) plan ahead. My favorite restaurants are ones that have their menus, with nutritional values, online. In my area these include Applebee's, Ruby Tuesday's, Panera's, Bob Evans, Olive Garden and Jose Peppers to mention a few. You can find nearly any restaurant by searching for "NAME OF RESTAURANT menu nutrition."

2) know without looking at a menu that anything with a cream sauce or butter or is fried or breaded is going to be high calorie and to be avoided. Better options are grilled or baked.

3) ask for condiments such as dressing for a salad, sour cream and butter for a baked potato to be brought on the side. Use just what you need as you eat rather than dumping the whole thing over the food. For salads, dip your fork in the dressing, then pick up a bite of salad. You get the flavor without more calories than are necessary.

4) share or ask for a to-go box. Portion sizes in restaurants are not realistic. The cheapest part of running a restaurant is the food and owners want you to think you are getting a good deal. Eating 2-3 times the portion size you need is not a good deal for the obese individual. Take 1/2 to 2/3 of the meal home for additional meals or share with a family member or friend.

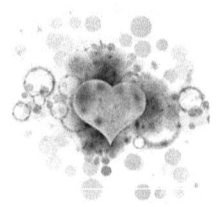

52: Personal chef?

I am probably one of the few people in the world who has never watched an Oprah television show. Toward the end I kind of wished I had, but I stopped watching TV after one that we had stopped working and found that it was a habit I didn't need to pick up again.

I have heard, however, about Oprah's weight loss efforts and I admire the way she was able to go online and air the problems that she encountered.

I would bet, though, that some of you, like me, found yourself thinking that if you could have a personal chef like Rosie Daley to plan, cook and present your meals that you wouldn't have any problem losing weight. Life, even weight loss, would be simple. After all, money will buy anything ... right?

Wrong! Money will buy more expensive food and someone to make life easier for you, but unless you are willing to take responsibility for your own weight loss it will not become something that you can do naturally for the rest of your life.

There are actually many companies, organizations and services now that will cook your meals and deliver them to your home—for a hefty price. But learning to cook your own meals easily, inexpensively is something that you will be able to fall back on the rest of your life.

Sharon Kay, M.A., L.U.T.

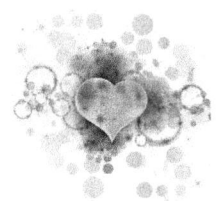

53: Health/Lifestyle Choices

There are two groups of people I would like to just grab and shake some sense into. One is the parents of overweight children. The other is morbidly obese individuals in wheelchairs.

In regard to the parents of overweight children, I do realize that very few people set out to ruin their children's lives. I know I did the same thing to my children and it certainly wasn't from a concept of wanting to destroy them. But I made a lot of misguided mistakes due to lack of knowledge on my part.

For example, I remember that my daughter loved raw vegetables when she was little and would often ask for a salad when eating out. Though we would buy her the salad, we also teased her unmercifully about being a "rabbit." Naturally, she worked to fit in and became, as an adult—guess what—morbidly obese.

Developing poor eating habits when you are young is a recipe for having problems all of your life. Most children could very easily be molded to healthy lifestyles if their parents were educated in how to eat properly themselves.

It is seldom a matter of not having the money to eat properly. A beans, rice and vegetables diet is very healthy if prepared properly. So many low income people, based on personal observations of women in crisis centers, go to corner convenience stores where food items cost 2-3 times as much as in grocery stories.

When I see a huge person in a wheelchair, with massive amounts of fat overhanging, I find it hard not to judge them. You know by my before photograph that I have been that large, though, by the grace of God, not wheelchair bound. There is no way that they are having any kind of quality life when they can't even walk to do their grocery shopping.

But if, as I believe, we attract our bodies by what we think about ourselves, these people have to be educated first in how to love themselves rather than in how to lose weight.

I was once told by a fitness coach to lovingly rub lotion onto my body, especially parts I didn't like, talking to those parts and telling them how much I love and appreciate them.

I do realize how difficult this is for the extremely large person to do and feel that they mean it. One of Unity's slogan, though, is "fake it 'til you make it" and I understand now how important that is. Saying we love our bodies just the way they are will create in us a subconscious effect of creating a body that we can love—without conscious effort.

As you make the decision to work seriously on losing weight you have two choices:

1) You can go into a plan with the idea of enjoying every minute, all day everyday, focusing on all of the good things that are happening to you, including eating foods you enjoy; or

2) You can begin your plan bitching every minute about how deprived you are. You can look at the person at the table next to you wolfing down a plateful of spaghetti with meatballs, garlic bread, salad drowning in high fat dressing and dessert... while you make the choice to have a meal that is 500 calories or less.

What you don't see, but have personally experienced yourself, is how the person feels after the meal is ended. They go home, sit down in front of the TV stomach hurting from the overindulgence, not feeling like any activity including sex and definitely not up to going out and having fun.

You, on the other hand, after a month of lovingly taking care of your body, will begin to have more energy, more interest in doing things that you used to do for fun, and in general will be enjoying your life and family.

What are you waiting for?

Last night a girlfriend and I went to a comedy club. We were seated on the front row. I ate a light meal at home before going and enjoyed a glass of chardonnay and nibbled on some nachos at the club.

As part of the show four members of the audience were asked to come on stage and participate. I was one of the ones chosen.

When I was at my maximum weight I would never have been chosen to come up on stage for several reasons—all hinging on the fact that an obese woman would not make a good participant. As it was, I had a great time and so did my friend.

What are you waiting for?

Sharon Kay, M.A., L.U.T.

The following is an excerpt from *Work Rules!* by (2015) Lazlo Bock, SVP of People Operations at Google. Bock discusses workplace changes Google implemented that enabled employees to cut three million calories from their diets. Google, which supplies all food and snacks for employees, made some minor changes that resulted in significantly less calorie intake by employees.

"In our Boulder, Colorado, office we measured the consumption of microkitchen snacks for two weeks to generate a baseline, and then put all the candy in opaque containers. Googlers, being normal people, prefer candy to fruit, but what would happen when we made the candy just a little less visible and harder to get to?

"We were floored by the result. The proportion of total calories consumed from candy decreased by 30 percent and the proportion of fat consumed dropped by 40 percent as people opted for the more visible granola bars, chips, and fruit. Heartened by the result, we did the same thing in our New York office. Healthy snacks like dried fruit and nuts were put in glass containers, and sweets were hidden in colored containers.

"After seven weeks, Googlers in our New York office had eaten 3.1 million (3,100,000!) fewer calories—enough to avoid gaining a cumulative 885-pounds."

Very impressive results and the type of change that you can make in your own home. Anything that should be eaten in limited quantities should be less accessible. Fruits and vegetables that can be eaten in virtually unlimited quantities should be front and center.

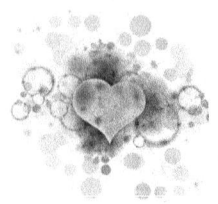

54: Strange dietary choices

My menu choices may sometimes seem strange to you, but probably no stranger than your can of SpaghettiOs now sounds to me (I actually had to do an internet search to be sure they still make these round circles in spaghetti sauce)!

Today, for example, I knew I had an evening event, but didn't know what or how much there would be to eat. It is OA, so I was sure there would be something I could eat. I chose to have a small lunch to keep my body from going into starvation mode. I

That mini-meal consisted of two slices of 45-calorie per slice bread with two thin slices of lunch meat and some asparagus spears I had already cooked in the refrigerator. For about 150 calories I had nutrients that were adequate to meet my body's immediate needs.

I have read that women in my age group, and I believe it could be generalized to other groups, do better eating six mini meals a day rather than three large meals. The idea is that our bodies can process small quantities much easier than they can process a system that is overloaded.

It is rather like what a doctor in my early years called an alley cat diet. He said, "Have you ever seen a fat alley cat?" Of course one thing he neglected to say was that those cats spend a lot of time running off the calories they consume!

Sharon Kay, M.A., L.U.T.

After reading this section I know that I am _____

_____

_____

_____

_____

_____

_____

_____

_____

_____

_____

_____

_____

_____

_____

_____

_____

_____

_____

_____

_____

_____

_____

PART SEVEN

Meals,

Menus

and More

The following section of photographs show actual meals I eat. The photography is not professional, but was done with my LG Optimus L70 cell phone. My goal is to present realism as opposed to "glamour" meals seen in magazines that make you salivate and run to the nearest store to purchase ingredients needed to prepare the recipes.

I chose seven representative days and included each day's menu and analysis of breakfasts, lunches and dinners. Many more will be offered on my website in the future. Understand that these 7 meals represent a variety of meals that I cook during a period of time.

Since I cook in quantity, I have multiple meals from each item that I cook for lunch and dinners Kama therefore, I eat the same thing several days in a row. For those of you who manage to live busy, hectic lifestyles, that is the only way practical to keep nutrition level in balance and still be able to enjoy your life without having to concentrate on cooking all the time—and without having to reach for fast food.

Each page includes a discussion of ingredients and preparation needed, points and the nutritional data that I use to calculate points, plus cost of the meal. Although I have an official Weight Watchers points calculator, there are acceptable online substitutes such as the following which purports to be equivalent to the Weight Watchers calculator:

http://www.calculatorcat.com/free_calculators/
weight_watchers_calculator.phtml

I make no claims as to the website's legality, but the calculator seems to be reasonably accurate. I would nevertheless encourage you to visit a Weight Watchers meeting and learn the program.

Making substitutions is easy. If you just can't stand any green vegetables (though I strongly encourage you to develop a taste for at least one green leafy vegetable because of the nutrients they provide and their low calorie content) replace them with orange carrots, yellow squash or purple eggplant.

It is very important that you do not just follow what I have written verbatim. Adjustments will need to be made for your current weight, gender, level of activity, allergies, etc.

A man trying to eat the quantities that I eat would probably feel like he was starving due to the fact that his metabolism burns more calories than does a woman's.

I don't like to think about what would happen if you are allergic to peanuts and eat my peanut butter and cherry sandwich for breakfast!

Please use common sense.

Sharon Kay, M.A., L.U.T.

Photographs are printed in grayscale due to prohibitive cost for color photographs. Color images would double the cost of the book and the intention is for it to be easily accessible to everyone who needs it. You can go to my website at www.SharonKays.website/color-booklet and browse or download a PDF of those pages.

The website also includes my blog, ways in which I can work with you or your group, links to tools you can use and much more. It will grow as your interest in my work grows. In other words, ask me questions. They will be answered. Invite me to do a workshop or retreat for your group, either at Unity Village or a location of your choosing. We will get acquainted personally and you will go away with many tools that you will use to create a happier, more healthy lifestyle.

I know that some of you, especially those of you who run into a fast food place for every meal, are telling yourself how impossible it would be to prepare meals that I describe. You don't have time. You don't know how to cook. You ... fill in the blank.

Today I came home from work at 3:30 p.m. and worked on the computer for about two hours. Then I:

1) prepared a package of just add water and milk Idahoan Applewood Smoked Bacon potatoes au gratin (25 minutes at 450°) and put them in the oven. (**NOTE:** I use almond milk and no margarine.)

2) when the potatoes were almost done I warmed a 3 oz. slice of deli ham in a dry skillet and microwave warmed broccoli I had cooked the day before.

3) put the three items on a 10 1/2" china plate (plates shown are not miniatures), sprayed the broccoli with butter flavored cooking spray and sprinkled it with salt.

Most of my meals require no more time or effort than this.

When you have a family or are entertaining, you simply warm additional slices of ham and increase the amount of broccoli.

If the quantities I eat are not sufficient to satisfy your hunger, don't hesitate to add servings of 0-point vegetables and fruit. In fact, a salad made with fat-free salad dressing and 0-point vegetables or a cup (or two) of 0-point vegetable soup before eating your main meal is a great idea. Just avoid adding high calorie items such as cheese, beans or croutons to a salad or pasta, beans or starchy vegetables to soup.

Numerous recipes for Weight Watchers 0-point soup can be found by doing an internet search for "0-point soup." Basically, I start with several cups of bouillon soup, a head of cabbage and an onion chopped, a can of tomatoes and spices (Mexican or Italian combinations are great). Bring to a boil. Then add 0-point vegetables you like.

NOTE: Potato mix makes five 1/2 cup servings. As soon as I take it out of the oven I portion the casserole into four individual bowls and one serving onto my plate. The additional four servings will be used during the week for lunches and dinners.

Sharon Kay, M.A., L.U.T.

The type meals you will see in the following pages will be served to you when you attend any of my retreats or workshops and each event will include one or more classes on cooking for health and releasing weight—on a budget! If you don't have to worry about making your dollars stretch father, just substitute more expensive meats and seafood.

As I've said before, cooking and eating should be fun experiences. They do not have to be difficult, nor do they have to be unhealthy.

I have just spent an evening with people who are vegetarian, students of macrobiotics, and would never consider eating the way that I propose in this book. However, for the person who weights 300-pounds or more, my suggestions represent a much healthier, balanced plan than they are accustomed to eating.

Take what resonates as truth for you and leave the rest. I suspect that the most diet-conscious reader can understand the importance of learning to love ourselves and treat our bodies with love and respect.

ADDENDUM 2a: Sample Day's Menu - Day 1

ITEM	CALORIES	BALANCE	POINTS	BALANCE
Any Date, Any Month 2015		1,200		32
Breakfast				
2 Live G free blueberry pancakes	-180	1,020	(4)	28
1 peach, sliced	-50	970	0	28
3 sl. precooked bacon	-105	865	(3)	25
1/2 C. almond milk	-15	850	0	25
1st Break				
1/4 C. blueberries & kiwi	-67	783	0	25
2nd Break				
1 C. cantaloupe	-60	723	0	25
Lunch				
1/4 C. Curly's BBQ Pulled Beef	-60	663	(3)	22
Delightful Hamburger bun	-80	583	(2)	20
Potato, yellow	-125	458	(4)	16
Dinner				
3 oz. deli ham	-120	338	(3)	13
1/2 C. potatoes au gratin (from mix)	-100	238	(4)	9
1 C. broccoli	-50	188	0	9
Coffee w/3T creamer / 5 tsp sugar	-120	68	(3)	6
3 Lemon thin cookies	-60	8	(3)	3

* I find calorie counts either on the food package (varies from brand to brand) or on the http://nutritiondata.self.com/ website.

NOTE: Nearly any recipe can be lightened to have less calories and/or points without sacrificing flavor or texture. If you have a favorite recipe and cannot figure out how to make it fit into your program, please write to me through my website and ask me if I have any suggestions for doing so.

Sharon Kay, M.A., L.U.T.

Blueberry Pancakes, Bacon and Peaches

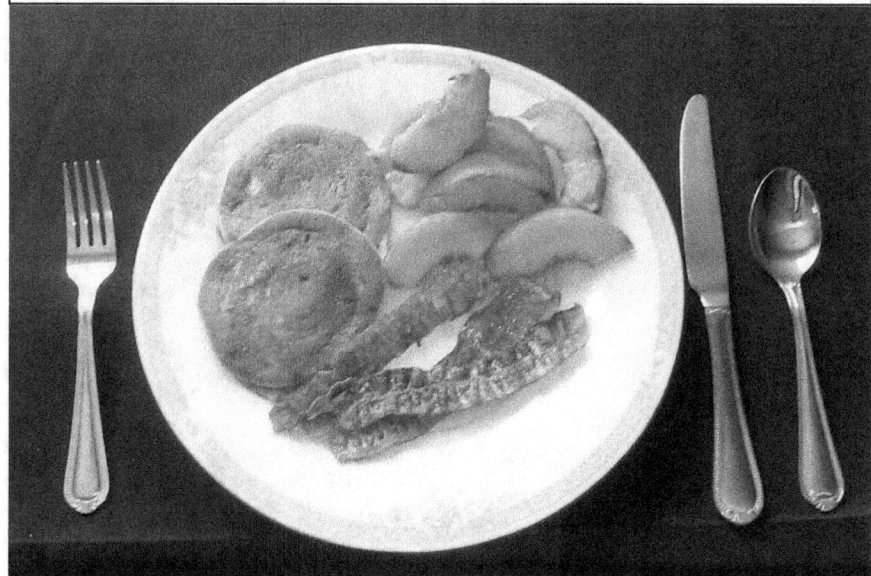

Frozen gluten-free blueberry pancakes with fresh peach slices and three slices precooked bacon. Ordinarily I would put one table-spoon real maple syrup on the pancakes but, because I planned my day's plan in advance I knew it would exceed my daily allowance.

Slice peach onto plate. Microwave pancakes on microwavable plate (my gold rim china is not) for 30-45 seconds (microwaves vary). Then microwave bacon for 25 seconds and your breakfast is ready.

This peach was tart. I could have sprinkled 1 tsp. raw sugar over it for 15 calories and 0 points, but I chose not to. Instead, be-cause eating the pancakes with syrup first would have made the tart-ness of the peach even more pronounced, I ate the peach first, then the pancakes and bacon.

I always add 1/2 cup vanilla almond milk (40 calories/0 points) and use this calcium rich drink to take a high-potency multiple vitamin and vitamin D3.

	Calories	Protein	Carbs	Fat	Fiber	Points	Cost
2 liveGfree frozen pancakes	160	4	26	4	1	4	0.50
3 sl. Farmland precooked bacon	90	7	0	6	0	3	1.00
Peach, fresh	59	1.4	14	0.4	2.2	0	0.25

Barbecue Shredded Beef with Potato Wedges

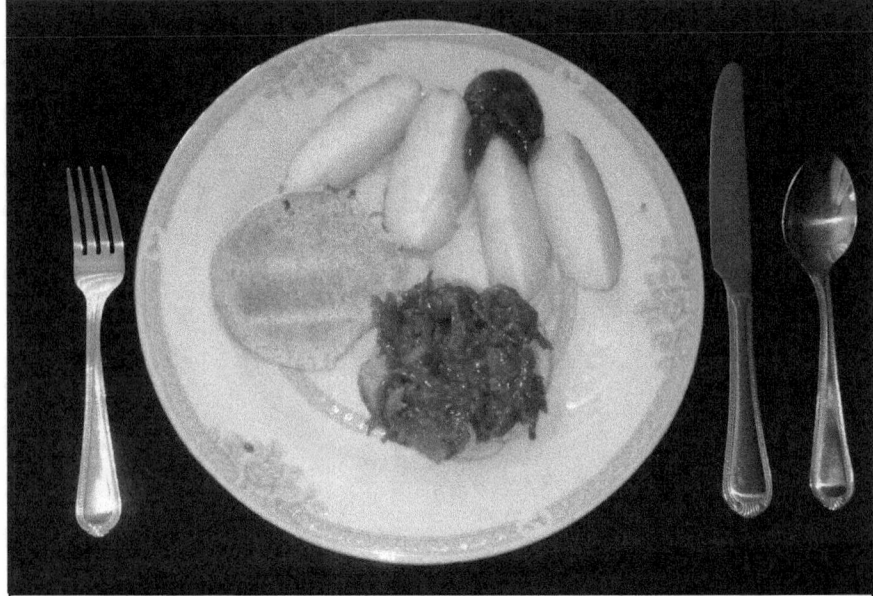

Curley's shredded barbecue beef or pork (beef has less calories) come prepackaged in the meat section of my grocery store. Warm 1/4 cup in the microwave and toast the bun while the potato is baking in the microwave for 3 minutes.

Serve with condiments - ketchup for the potato and optional onion and dill pickle spears (not shown).

	Calories	Protein	Carbs	Fat	Fiber	Points	Cost
1/4 C. Curly's BBQ Pulled Beef	-60	4	14	2	1	3	0.50
Delightful Hamburger bun	-80	4	20	0.5	7	2	0.15
Potato, yellow	-130	3	30	0	3	4	0.10

Sharon Kay, M.A., L.U.T.

Ham, Au Gratin Potatoes and Broccoli

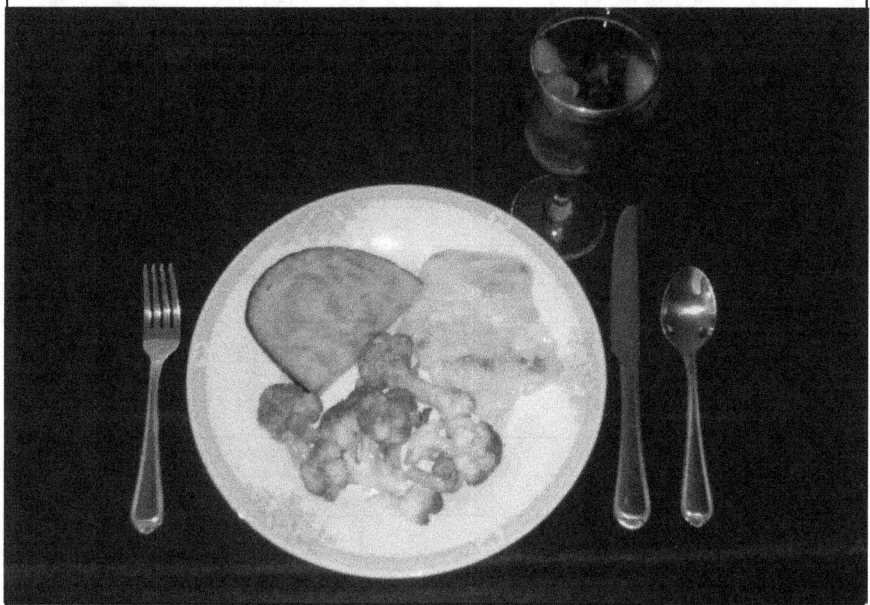

Lean, 98% fat-free, slices of ham from the deli section at your grocery store provide high quality protein and are quick and easy to warm in a dry pan on top of the stove or in a microwave.

When I got home from work I mixed a box of potatoes au gratin according to the directions on the box, but using almond milk and no added fat. They baked 25 minutes and I let them sit for 30 minutes giving the cheese sauce time to thicken.

Broccoli cooked the day before took 1 minute to warm in the microwave.

	Calories	Protein	Carbs	Fat	Fiber	Points	Cost
3 oz. Black Forest deli ham	-120	15	2	2	0	3	1.25
1 C. broccoli, cooked	-50	4	10	1	4	0	0.25
1/2 C. potatoes au gratin	-100	2	21	1	1	3	0.25

ADDENDUM 2b: Sample Day's Menu - Day 2

ITEM	CALORIES	BALANCE	POINTS	BALANCE
Any Date, Any Month 2015		1,200		32
Breakfast				
45 gr. Special K w/red berries	-165	1,035	(5)	27
3 T. fat-free coffee creamer	-30	1,005	(1)	26
1/2 C. almond milk	-15	990	0	26
1 C. honeydew melon	-60	930	0	26
1st Break				
Apple	-50	880	0	26
2nd Break				
1/2 C. grapes	-52	828	0	26
Lunch				
2 oz. Buddig, thin beef	-90	738	(2)	24
Sara Lee Delightful bun	-80	658	(2)	22
Lettuce, tomato, mayo/mustard	-10	648	0	22
1 medium potato (2"x3")	-125	523	(4)	18
Dinner				
5 oz. pork loin slice	-220	303	(6)	12
Mushroom, Onion, Garlic	-50	253	0	12
Corn-on-the-Cob	-90	163	(3)	9
Coffee w/3T creamer / 5 tsp sugar	-120	43	(3)	6
2 Lemon thin cookies	-40	3	(3)	3

Sharon Kay, M.A., L.U.T.

Special K Cereal with Berries

and Honeydew Melon

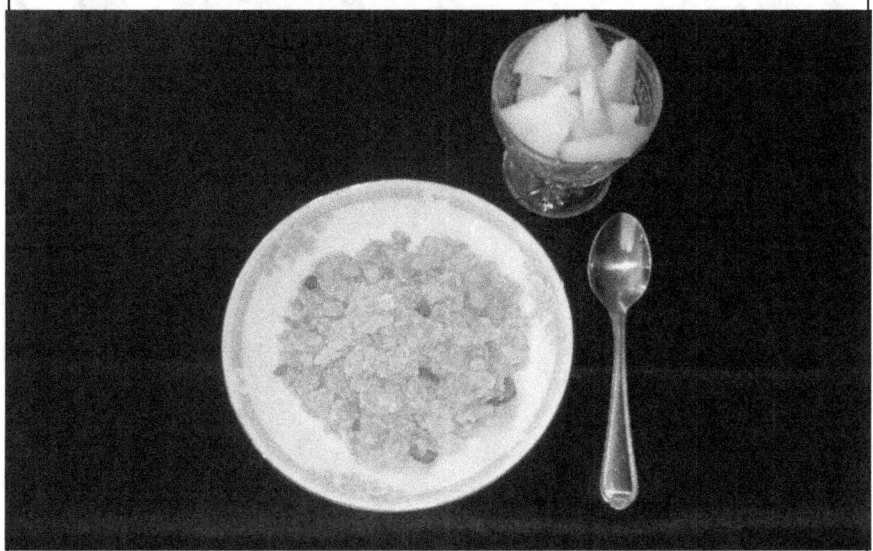

Special K cereals have come to be my favorite dry breakfast cereal. I usually keep 2-3 different flavors on-hand. The one shown is Special K with Red Berries (dried strawberries). Another favorite is Cinnamon Pecan. They are sweet, crunchy and filling. I do find that the serving size of 3/4 to 1 cup is not enough for me. I have 1 1/8 to 1 1/2 cups (45 grams). It is easy in getting ready for work to put a bowl on my scale, weigh 45 grams of cereal and top it with 45 grams (three tablespoons) coffee creamer.

I have my 1/2 cup almond milk with the cereal before going to work.

The breakfast shown was on a Saturday and I added one cup of honeydew chunks—which were from one of the sweetest melons I have ever eaten!

	Calories	Protein	Carbs	Fat	Fiber	Points	Cost
45 gr. Special K w/red berries	165	3	41	0	4.5	4	1.25
3 T. coffee creamer	45	0	3	3	0	1	0.25
1/2 C. almond milk	20	0.5	1	1.5	0.5	0	0.25
1 C. honeydew melon	60	1	16	0	1	0	0.35

Thin Beef Sandwich with Mock Fries

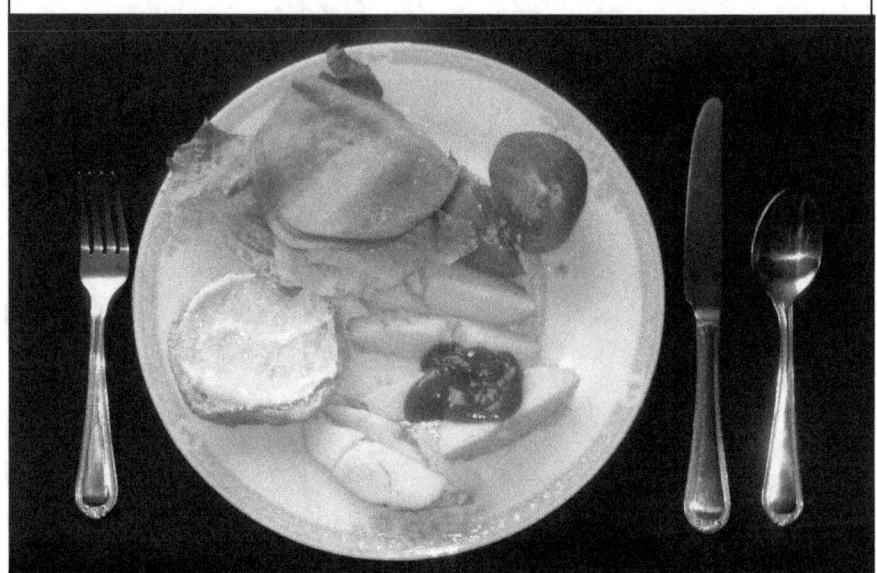

My evening meal is often a sandwich on Sara Lee Delightful hamburger bun or bread slices. This meal, which was a Saturday lunch instead of dinner, consisted of thin sliced beef (two ounces of any thin sliced luncheon meat would be fine), Sara Lee Delightful hamburger bun spread with a mixture of fat-free Kraft mayonnaise and mustard, plus lettuce and sliced fresh homegrown tomato.

The potato was baked in a microwave for three minutes, sliced, salted and served with ketchup. And, yes, you could have an equivalent number of calories in potato chips. But remember that they won't keep hunger at bay as long—and what do you do with the remainder of the bag of chips?

	Calories	Protein	Carbs	Fat	Fiber	Points	Cost
2 oz. Buddig thin beef	90	10	1	5	0	2	0.50
Sara Lee Delightful bun	80	4	20	0.5	7	2	0.35
Lettuce, tomato, mayo/mustard	10	INSIGNIFICANT AMOUNTS				0	0.05
1 medium potato (2"x3")	163	0	37	2	4.7	4	0.10

Sharon Kay, M.A., L.U.T.

Roast Pork Loin with Mushrooms, Onions, Garlic Cloves and Corn-On-the-Cob

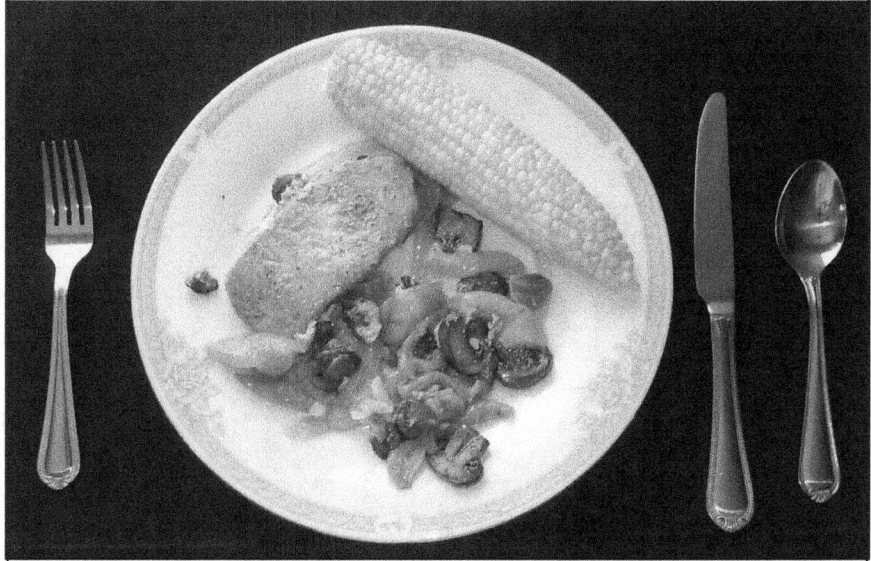

It would be difficult to get much easier than this meal.

Nine precut, pre-weighed (five ounces each) pork loin slices were put in the bottom of a roasting pan, sprinkled with salt and pepper, turned over and additional salt and pepper sprinkled on the second side.

A one-pound package of pre-sliced baby bella mushrooms was layered on top of the pork with five yellow onions cut in wedges and three bulbs of peeled, sliced garlic, with additional salt and pepper. (Other favorite spices optional.)

Meat and vegetables were slow roasted (350∘) for 1 1/2 hours.

Serve with corn-on-the cob microwaved on high for four minutes, sprayed with Parkay 0-calorie spray and sprinkled with salt and pepper.

	Calories	Protein	Carbs	Fat	Fiber	Points	Cost
5 oz. pork loin slice	220	25	0	12.5	0	6	1.50
Mushroom, Onion, Garlic	50	3	8	0	3	0	0.75
Corn-on-the-Cob	90	3	19	1	1	3	0.25

ADDENDUM 2c: Sample Day's Menu—Day 3

ITEM	CALORIES	BALANCE	POINTS	BALANCE
Any Day, Any Month, 2016		1,200		32
Breakfast				
2 sl. Sara Lee Delightful bread	-90	1,110	(2)	30
1 T. peanut butter	-90	1,020	(3)	27
10 Cherries	-50	970	0	27
1/2 C. almond milk	-15	955	0	27
1st Break				
1 C. cantaloupe	-60	895	0	27
2nd Break				
Peach	-50	845	0	27
Lunch				
Stouffer's stuffed pepper	-190	705	(5)	22
1/2 C. potatoes au gratin	-100	605	(4)	18
1 C. zucchini	-35	570	0	18
Dinner				
Chicken Cordon Bleu	-230	340	(6)	12
Spinach & 6 T. egg substitute	-95	245	(1)	11
2/3 C. corn	-70	175	(3)	8
Coffee w/3T creamer / 5 tsp sugar	-120	55	(3)	5
3 lemon thins	-60	(5)	(2)	3

Sharon Kay, M.A., L.U.T.

Peanut Butter Sandwich with Black Cherries

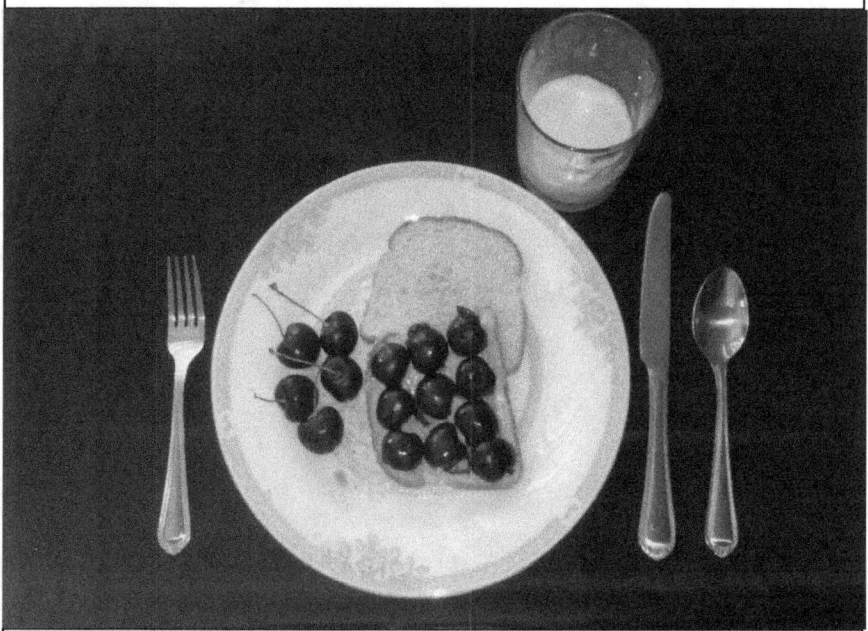

As those of you with children can attest, nothing is easier for breakfast than a peanut butter and jelly sandwich. This version is a bit more grown-up and requires pitting cherries—but is well worth the effort when the cherries are big, fresh and sweet.

If you are just beginning your weight loss efforts you may find this to be a "snack" rather than a breakfast. In that case, have two sandwiches. You will notice that it only took half (5) of the cherries to cover the peanut butter. Have an open-face sandwich with 1 T. peanut butter on each slice. Just remember to count the extra peanut butter.

Play with your food! Figure out what works for you. After this "mini-breakfast" I go straight to work and take my mind off food. 1 to 1 1/2 hours later I have a piece of fruit. A second piece of fruit between then and my 1:30 lunch schedule usually satisfies me.

	Calories	Protein	Carbs	Fat	Fiber	Points	Cost
1 T. peanut butter	100	3.5	3	8	1	3	0.05
2 sl. Sara Lee Delightful bread	90	5	19	1	5	2	0.15
10 black cherries	50	1	12	0	2	0	0.55
1/2 C. almond milk (40 cal/cup)	20	0.5	1	1.5	0.5	0	0.14

Stuffed Bell Pepper, Zucchini and Potatoes au Gratin

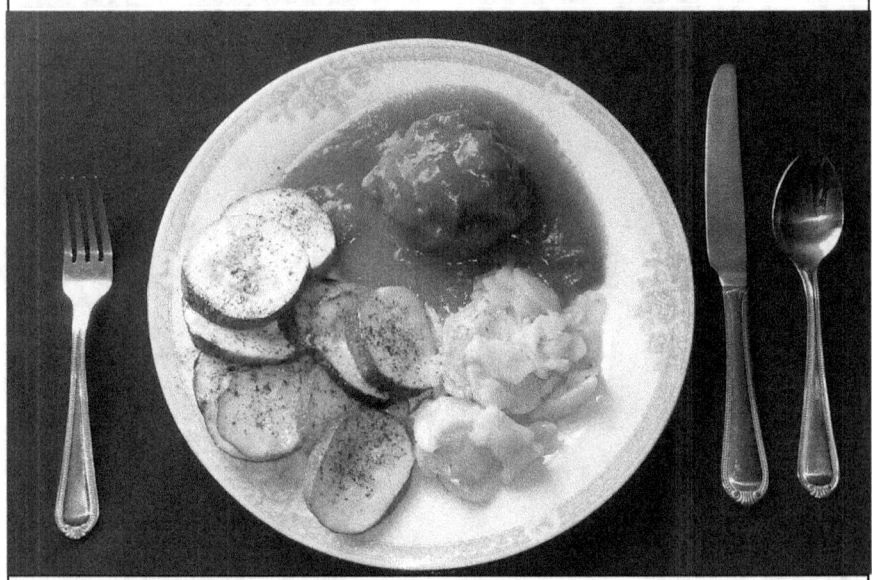

Frozen Stouffer stuffed bell peppers, which I choose to bake in a regular oven (though they are microwaveable), require 52 minutes to bake.

Boxed potatoes au gratin usually take 25 minutes, so pop them in the oven when the bell peppers are about 1/2 cooked.

I slice a zucchini, microwave it in a plastic bag and put in on the plate when meet and potatoes are ready. Spray with butter-flavored cooking spray and sprinkle with your favorite spices. Salt, pepper and chili powder are my favorites.

NOTE: There are four stuffed bell peppers in the package. The other three are put into my glass bowls with lids for either lunch or dinner meals that week.

	Calories	Protein	Carbs	Fat	Fiber	Points	Cost
Stouffer's stuffed pepper	190	8	21	7	4	5	2.00
1/2 C. potatoes au gratin	100	2	20	1.5	2	4	0.25
1 C. zucchini	35	2.5	6	0.5	2	0	0.30

Sharon Kay, M.A., L.U.T.

Chicken Cordon Bleu, Corn and Spinach with Egg

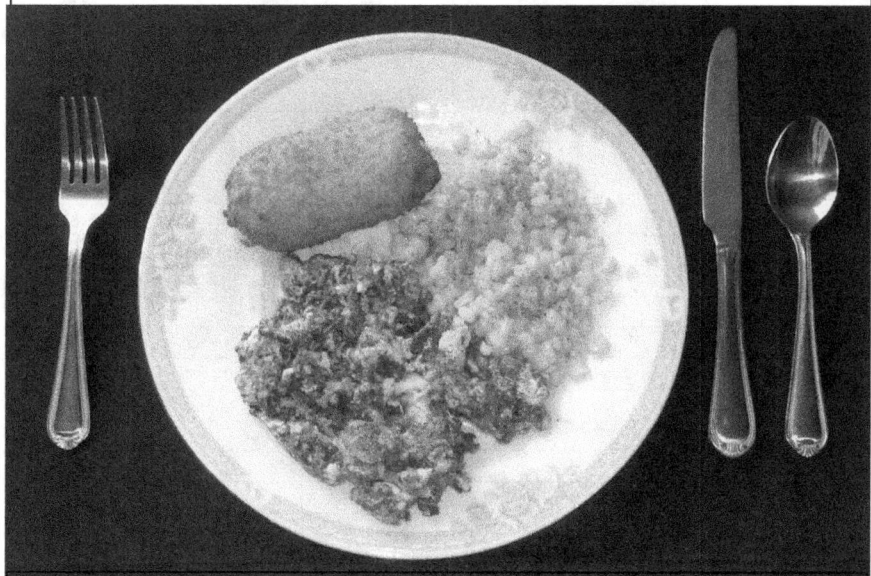

Frozen chicken cordon bleu, which must be baked in a regular oven, requires 25 minutes to bake.

Drain one can of spinach well. Sauté in 1 tsp. coconut oil until spinach is almost dry. Create a well in center of spinach, pour in 1/2 cup Egg Beaters or equivalent egg substitute and cook egg until set. Combine spinach and egg mixture. Sprinkle with salt and pepper, to taste. (Serves 2)

Thaw 2/3 cup corn kernels in microwave until hot. Spray with 0-point cooking spray and sprinkle with salt and pepper.

	Calories	Protein	Carbs	Fat	Fiber	Points	Cost
Chicken Cordon Bleu	-230	19	18	12	2	6	0.99
Spinach & 6 T. egg substitute	-95	8.5	7	0	3.5	1	0.80
2/3 C. corn	-70	3	21	1	1	3	0.30

ADDENDUM 2d: Sample Day's Menu—Day 4

ITEM	CALORIES	BALANCE	POINTS	BALANCE
Any Day, Any Month, 2016		1,200		32
Breakfast		1,200		32
Breakfast Bowl:		1,200		32
2 oz. thin ham, diced	-90	1,110	(2)	30
6 T. egg substitute	-50	1,060	(1)	29
1/2 oz. cheddar cheese, grated	-55	1,005	(2)	27
Potato, medium	-163	842	(4)	23
1/2, C. almond milk	-15	827	0	23
1st Break		827		23
Orange	-50	777	0	23
2nd Break		827		23
1 C. cantaloupe	-60	767	0	23
Lunch		767		23
3 oz. Smithfield smoked chops	-110	657	(3)	20
10 asparagus spears	-30	627	0	20
1/2, C. baked acorn squash	-60	567	0	20
1 T. raw sugar w/butter spray	-45	522	(1)	19
Dinner		522		19
Tuna salad sandwich	-250	272	(4)	15
1/2, C. baked acorn squash	-60	212	0	15
Coffee w/3T creamer / 5 tsp sugar	-120	92	(3)	12

Sharon Kay, M.A., L.U.T.

Ham, Egg, Cheese
and Potato Breakfast Bowl

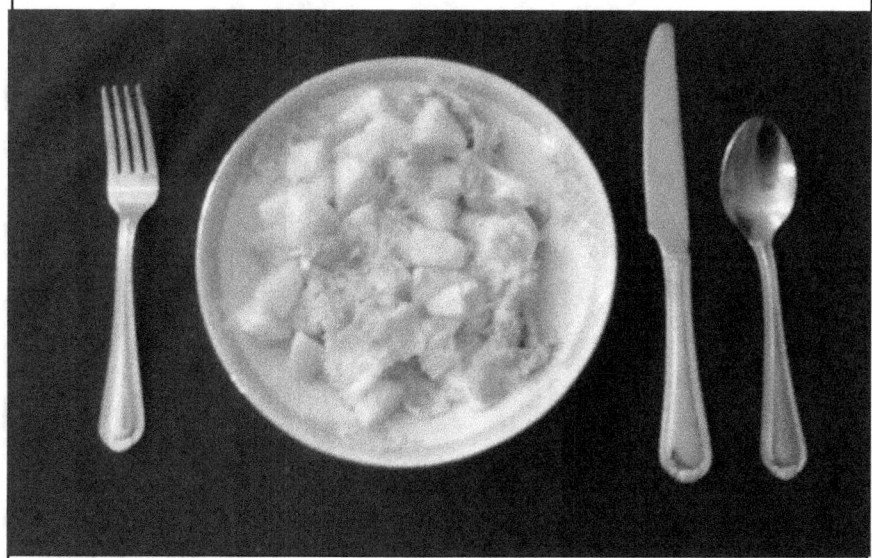

Bake potato in plastic bag in microwave 4 minutes, or until tender. Spray non-stick skillet with butter-flavored spray. Scramble egg substitute. Stir in ham. Two-ounces of any lean ham, such as deli ham, can be used. Cut potato into bite size pieces and stir into mixture. Sprinkle grated cheese on top and microwave 30 seconds to melt cheese.

(**NOTE:** Onion could be cooked in skillet before scrambling eggs for no additional points and few calories.)

This would be a good recipe to multiply times 2-4 servings. Divide portions into refrigerator containers. Warm in microwave for breakfasts, or even a fast evening meal.

	Calories	Protein	Carbs	Fat	Fiber	Points	Cost
2 oz. Buddig thin ham	90	10	1	5	0	2	0.50
6 T. egg substitute	80	5	<1	0	0	1	0.50
1/2 oz. cheddar cheese, grated	55	3.5	<1	9	0	0	0.15
1 medium potato (2"x3")	163	0	37	2	4.7	4	0.10

Smoked Pork Loin, Asparagus and Acorn Squash

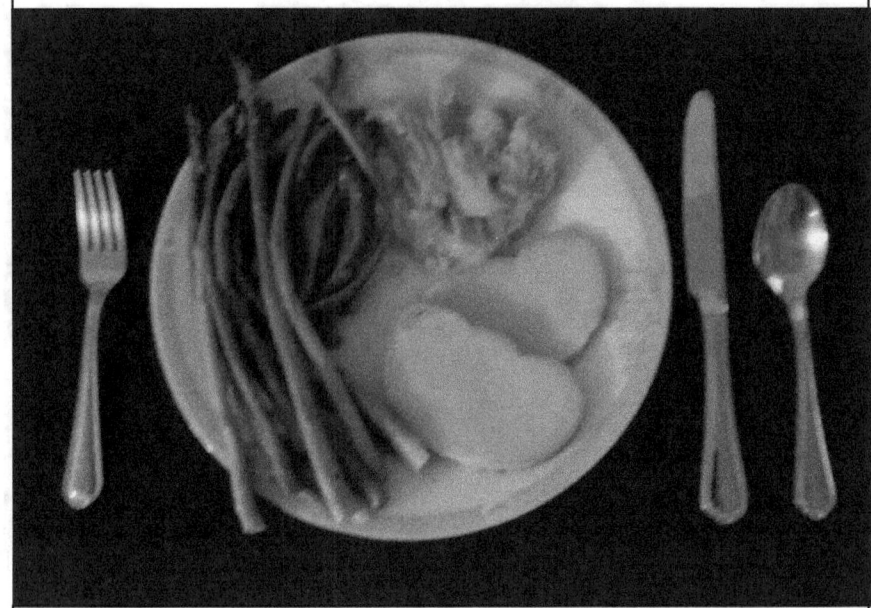

Smithfield pork loin slices (or pork chops) come precooked and sliced. All you need to do is warm the slices in a microwave or in a dry skillet at medium heat.

Steam 1-pound of asparagus in a plastic bag in microwave. Spray 10 stalks with butter-flavored cooking spray and sprinkle with salt, if desired.

Bake a large acorn squash in plastic bag in microwave for 6-10 minutes. Cut in half. Scoop out pulp and mash. Spray with cooking spray. (NOTE: Sometimes it's better to taste 0-point vegetables to see if they need any points added. I put sugar in this squash; then tasted a bite without sugar. It really need it unless you want a rich dessert.)

	Calories	Protein	Carbs	Fat	Fiber	Points	Cost
3 oz. Smithfield smoked chops	110	15	4	3.5	0	3	1.44
10 asparagus spears	30	4	6	0	3	0	0.40
1/2 C. baked acorn squash	60	1	8	0	1	0	0.30

Sharon Kay, M.A., L.U.T.

Tuna Salad Sandwich
with Sugar-Free Pickle Spears

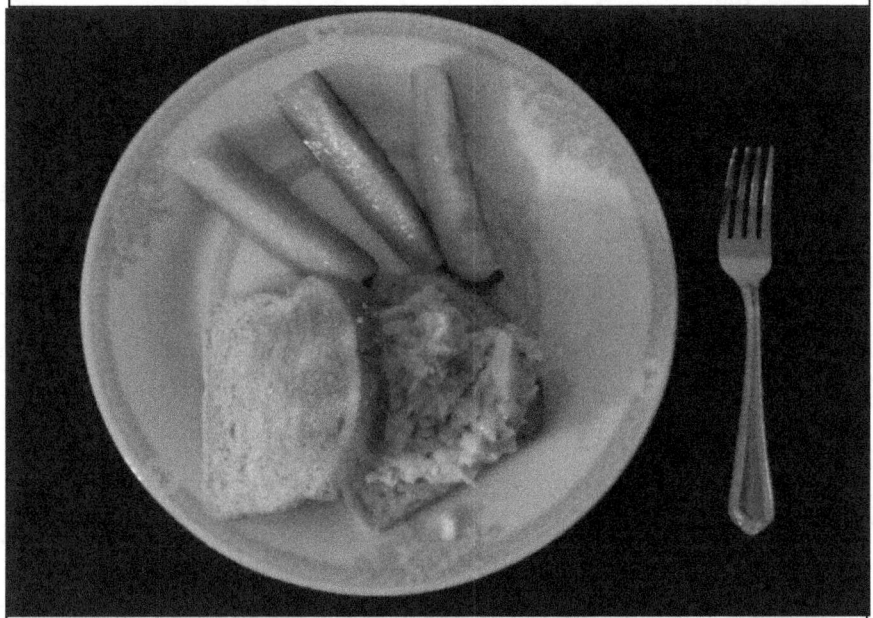

Tuna salad has never been one of my favorite sandwich fillings, but it is a good choice for releasing weight. With two slices of toasted Delightful bread this was quite good.

This evening I used an entire 5 oz. can of tuna packed in oil (in water would have been a few less calories, but, to be honest, I bought the wrong kind when it was on sale. I added 2 T. fat-free mayonnaise, 1/4 cup chopped onion (use as much as you like) and ate sugar-free bread 'n butter pickles on the side (again, eat as many as you like).

You may not be able to tell from the photograph, but this was a *lot* of tuna salad! It would have been sufficient for two sandwiches, but I preferred to just eat some of it with a fork.

I added corn squash, *without* sugar, for dessert.

	Calories	Protein	Carbs	Fat	Fiber	Points	Cost
Tuna salad	160	11	2	3	0	2	0.89
2 sl. Sara Lee Delightful bread	90	5	19	1	5	2	0.15
1/2 C. baked acorn squash	60	1	8	0	1	0	0.30

ADDENDUM 2e: Sample Day's Menu—Day 5

ITEM	CALORIES	BALANCE	POINTS	BALANCE
Any Day, Any Month, 2016		1,200		32
Breakfast				
Bread pudding	-263	937	(6)	26
1/2 C. almond milk	-15	922	0	26
		922		26
		922		26
1st Break				
C. cantaloupe	-60	862	0	26
2nd Break				
Orange	-50	812	0	26
Lunch				
3 oz. Beef fajitas, pre-cooked	-120	742	(3)	23
1/2 C. mixed greens w/bacon	-70	672	(2)	21
1 potato, mashed	-175	497	(4)	17
Dinner				
Vindaloo chicken thigh	-220	277	(7)	10
1 C. Bhindi masala (okra)	-50	227	(1)	9
1/2 C. white rice, cooked	-103	124	(3)	6
Coffee w/3T creamer / 5 tsp sugar	-120	4	(3)	3

Sharon Kay, M.A., L.U.T.

Bread Pudding

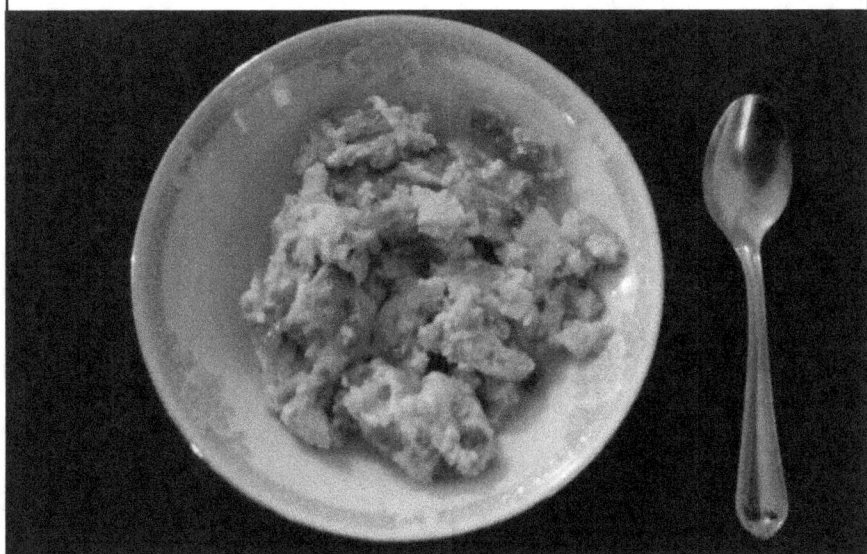

Few desserts are harder for me to resist than warm, home-made bread pudding. This recipe is a lighter version that I developed myself—and it cooks in the microwave in about 3-minutes!

Combine 3 tablespoons egg substitute with 1/2 cup almond milk. Add 1/2 teaspoon nutmeg (or cinnamon), dash of salt and 2 tablespoons raw sugar. Beat with whisk until well mixed. Cut, or break, two slices Sara Lee Delightful bread into small pieces and still into the milk mixture. Drop in 1/2-ounce raisins, distributing them evenly over surface. Pour into microwaveable bowl that holds about three times the amount of liquid (it boils over easily). Microwave on high for 1-minute. Stir. Repeat, as needed.

	Calories	Protein	Carbs	Fat	Fiber	Points	Cost
3 T. egg substitute	25	2.5	0	0	0	0	0.25
1/2 c. almond milk	15	0.5	1	1.5	0.5	0	0.25
1/2 tsp. nutmeg (or cinnamon)	0	0	0	0	0	0	0.00
Dash salt	0	0	0	0	0	0	0.00
2 T. raw sugar	90	0	24	0	0	3	0.05
2 sl. Sara Lee Delightful bread	90	5	19	1	5	2	0.15
1/2 oz. raisins	43	0.5	11	0	0.5	1	0.30

Beef Fajitas, Greens and Mashed Potatoes

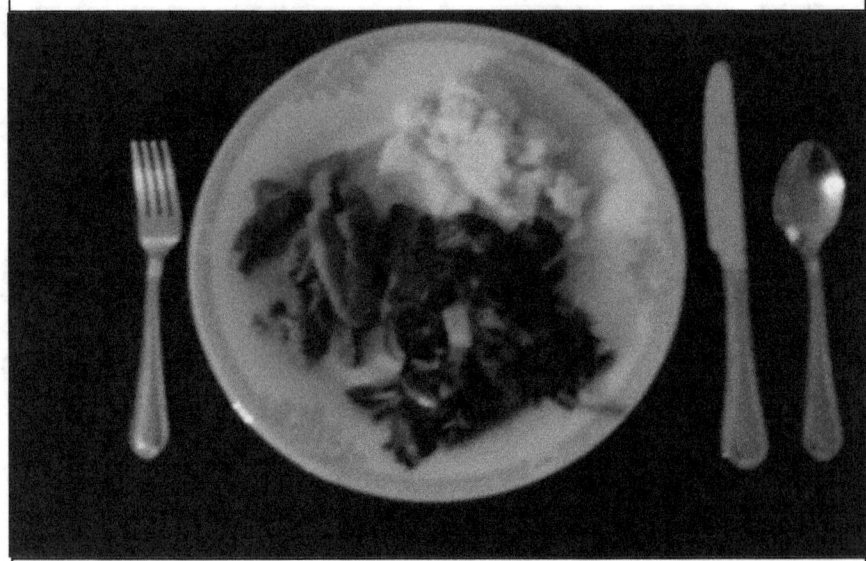

Put one-pound bag pre-washed green (collard, turnip, mustard or a mix) into 3-quart pan. Sprinkle one tablespoon raw sugar over greens, plus salt and pepper, if desired. Use kitchen shears to cut five slices of pre-cooked bacon into small strips over greens. Turn burner onto medium and cook for about 30 minutes, stirring occasionally, until desired tenderness.

Cook potato in microwave until soft. Peel, spray with butter-flavored cooking spray, sprinkle with salt and pepper, and mash with one tablespoon fat-free coffee creamer until creamy.

Warm pre-cooked fajita beef slices in microwave 30 seconds.

	Calories	Protein	Carbs	Fat	Fiber	Points	Cost
3 oz. Beef fajitas, pre-cooked	120	16	2	4.5	0	3	1.99
1/2 C. mixed greens w/bacon	70	4	17	2	3	2	0.65
1 potato, mashed	175	0	37	2	4.7	4	0.15

Sharon Kay, M.A., L.U.T.

Indian Vindaloo Chicken,
Bhindi Masala and Rice

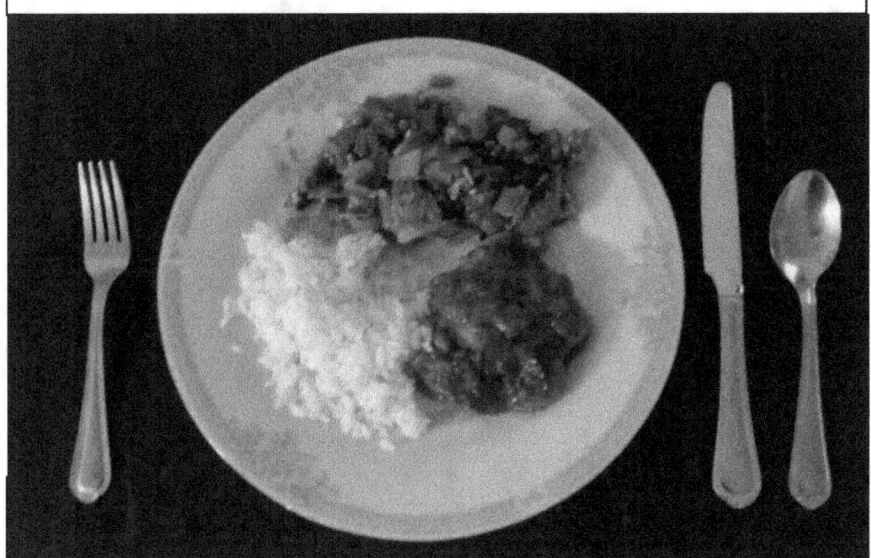

Vindaloo chicken is very labor intensive and costly—if you make homemade. Jars of Indian simmer sauces are readily available and very acceptable substitutes. Spread half a jar of sauce over bottom of rectangular baking dish, layout 4-6 boneless, skinless chicken thighs (1/2 breasts if you prefer), and spoon remaining sauce over top of chicken. Bake at 350° for 1 hour or until done.

Bhindi masala is my favorite Indian dish and is *very* weight loss friendly. The only ingredient counted as points is the coconut oil. Stir-fry chopped onion and two diced Roma tomatoes in four teaspoons coconut oil in large pot until onion is tender. Add two 12-ounce packages frozen okra. Sprinkle with two tablespoons garam masala, one teaspoon chili powder, and 1/2 teaspoon red pepper flakes (optional). adjusting spices to taste as okra cooks. Cook on medium high heat until okra is done. Remove lid and continue cooking until dish is fairly dry.

Serve with cooked white rice.

	Calories	Protein	Carbs	Fat	Fiber	Points	Cost
4 oz. chicken thigh, no skin/bone	130	22	0	4.5	0	4	1.01
1/3 C. Vindaloo simmer sauce	90	2	17	9	3	3	0.60
1 C. Bhindi masala	50	1	6	4	2	1	0.35
1/2 C. rice, white, cooked	103	2	23	0.2	0.3	3	0.10

ADDENDUM 2f: Sample Day's Menu—Day 6

ITEM	CALORIES	BALANCE	POINTS	BALANCE
Any Day, Any Month, 2016		1,200		32
Breakfast - 6:30 a.m.		1,200		32
9 T. scrambled egg substitute	-75	1,125	(1)	31
2 Jimmy Dean Maple Sausage	-110	1,015	(3)	28
2 T. picante sauce	-10	1,005	0	28
2 sl. Sara Lee Delightful bread	-90	915	(2)	26
1 T. Smucker's Simply Fruit	-40	875	(1)	25
1st Break		875		25
1 C. fresh pineapple	-82	793	0	25
2nd Break		793		25
1 C. cantaloupe	-60	815	0	25
Lunch		815		25
Banquet Cheesy Rice & Chicken	-190	625	(5)	20
1 C. mixed greens with bacon	-70	555	(2)	18
Dinner - 6:00 p.m.		555		18
Romaine lettuce	-10	545	0	18
Grilled chicken	-180	365	(3)	15
Fajita vegetables	-20	345	(3)	12
Black beans	-120	225	0	12
Tomatilla/green chili salsa	-15	210	0	12
Guacamole	-230	(20)	(6)	6

Sharon Kay, M.A., L.U.T.

Scrambled Eggs with Picante Sauce, Sausage Patties, Toast and Jam

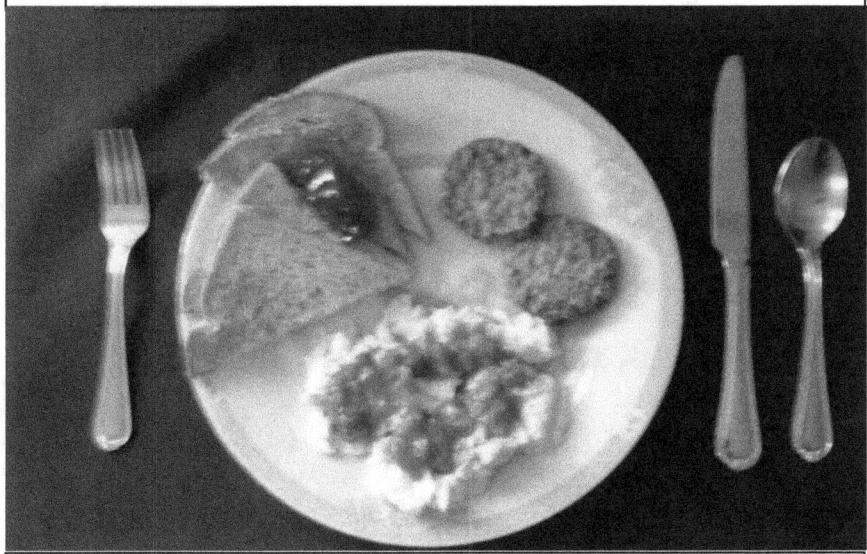

Scrambled egg substitute with two tablespoons picante sauce, two Jimmy Dean maple sausage patties and two slices Sara Lee Delightful bread, toasted with one tablespoon Smucker's Simply Fruit jam make a quick and easy breakfast.

I have been known to eat this, or a similar meal, for dinner. As you may remember, breakfasts were nearly the only meal my mother cooked and it is still my favorite meal of the day.

	Calories	Protein	Carbs	Fat	Fiber	Points	Cost
9 T. scrambled egg substitute	75	15	1	0	0	1	0.75
2 Jimmy Dean Maple Sausage	110	11	2	6	0	3	0.92
2 T. picante sauce	10	0	2	0	0	0	0.05
2 sl. Sara Lee Delightful bread	90	5	19	1	5	2	0.15
1 T. Smucker's Simply Fruit	40	0	10	0	0	1	0.15

DRESS UP A TV DINNER
Cheesy Rice and Chicken with Greens

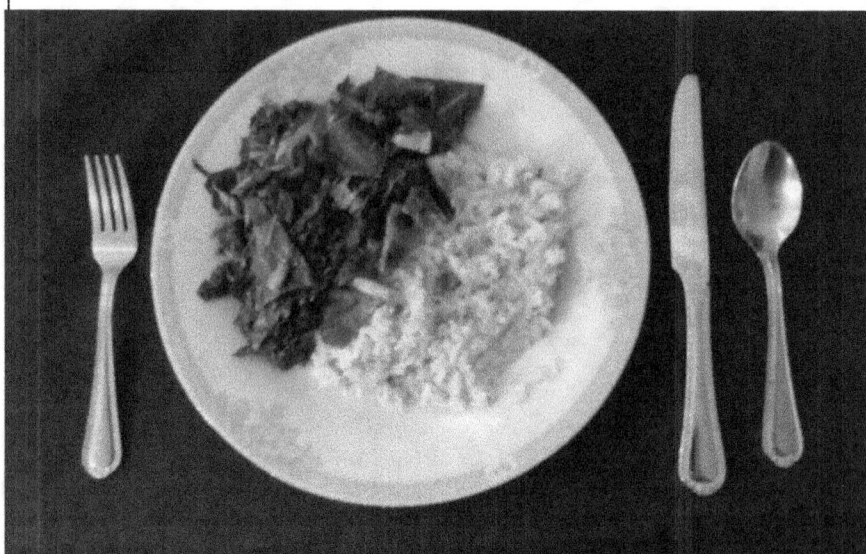

Several varieties of TV dinner are very reasonably price and, with the addition of a cooked vegetable or salad, can make a satisfying meal. The Cheesy Rice & Chicken shown is by Banquet and the regular price is $1.00. On sale you can frequently buy them 10/$8.00.

This meal has 8 grams of protein, 3 grams of fiber and is fairly low in sodium, making it a good choice.

Ordinarily I would have added additional broccoli, but I had the greens already cook—and they are so good!

I fixed this for lunch on a day that I had had almost back-to-back meetings the day before.

	Calories	Protein	Carbs	Fat	Fiber	Points	Cost
Banquet Cheesy Rice & Chicken	190	8	28	4.5	3	5	1.00
1 C. mixed greens with bacon	70	4	17	2	3	2	0.65

DINING OUT: *Chipotle Restaurant Salad and Salsa*

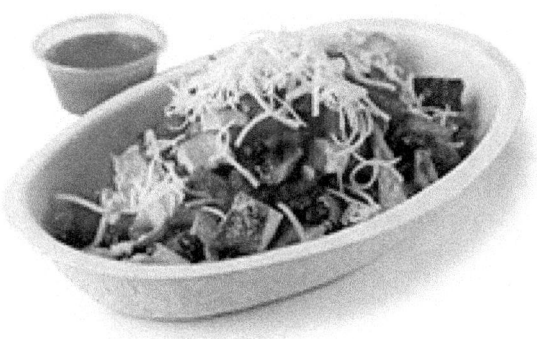

Chipotle Restaurant is one of the most health conscious, weight loss friendly places to eat in our area. In addition, all ingredients are guaranteed to be fresh and organic.

I went to a friend's art gallery showing this afternoon *and*, bonus, I had received in the mail a coupon for a free salad, burrito or tacos at Chipotle. Free is always a nice enticement for me!

The photograph shown is from their website so my bowl didn't look exactly like this one, but you can go to their website at www.chipotle.com and build your own salad before you leave home.

I had a bed of romaine lettuce topped with chicken, fajita vegetables, black beans, tomatillo green chili salsa and guacamole. Doing without the guacamole would have been less calories and points, but I love guacamole, it's an excellent fat source and I used it in place of their salad dressing which would have had as many calories and no nutrient value.

Notice that 120 calories (about 1/2 cup) of beans was 0-points. That's because of the 12-grams of fiber!

	Calories	Protein	Carbs	Fat	Fiber	Points	Cost
Romaine lettuce	10	0	2	0	1	0	0.00
Grilled chicken	180	32	0	7	0.5	3	0.00
Fajita vegetables	20	1	22	0.5	1	3	0.00
Black beans	120	7	4	1	12	0	0.00
Tomatilla/green chili salsa	15	0	4	0	0	0	0.00
Guacamole	230	2	8	22	6	6	0.00

ADDENDUM 2g: Sample Day's Menu—Day 7

ITEM	CALORIES	BALANCE	POINTS	BALANCE
Any Day, Any Month, 2016		1,200		32
Breakfast - 6:30 a.m.		1,200		32
Vegetable Omelet	-290	910	(7)	25
3 sl. bacon	-140	770	(4)	21
Scrambled Egg Whites	-50	720	(1)	20
Fruit Dish	-45	675	0	20
Lunch		675		20
1/4 Bremer lasagna w/meat sauce	-220	455	(6)	14
0-point fresh vegetables	-30	425	0	14
2 T. blue cheese dressing	-130	295	(4)	10
Dinner - 6:00 p.m.		455		14
Petite sirloin (7 oz.)	-365	90	(9)	5
Roasted spaghetti squash	-41	49	(1)	4
Grilled Zucchini	-54	(5)	(1)	3

This was a special day. Note that I ate both breakfast and dinner at restaurants without going over my daily limits significantly. In order to do so I skipped extra fruit and my nightly coffee and cookies. But I was with friends for the meals and it was worth it.

Sharon Kay, M.A., L.U.T.

DINING OUT: *Bob Evans*
Vegetable Omelet and Mixed Fruit

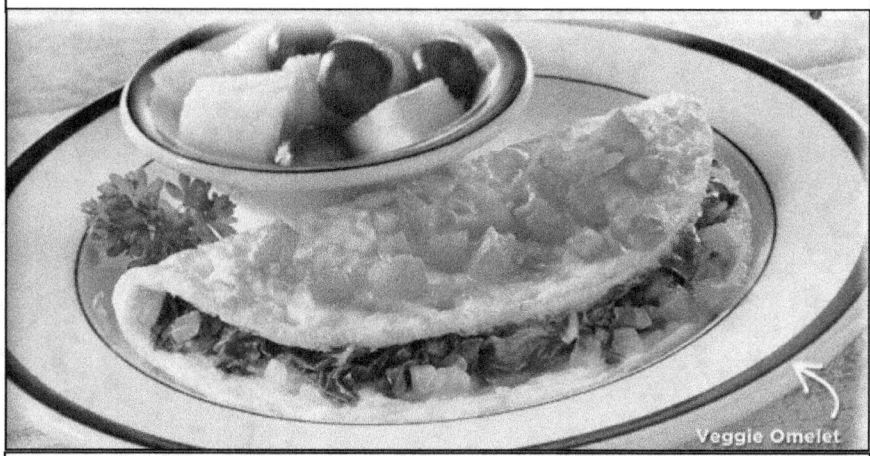

Veggie Omelet

Bob Evans restaurant is a favorite for a friend and me after an Overeater's Anonymous meeting. They have a wide range of options, serve breakfast all day, and information on nutrition is available on their website. In the menu, weight loss friendly items are "Fit From the Farm" selections.

This vegetable omelet, with a side order of fruit, is a good choice. Actually, you can add home fries and bacon without going off your program so I have included them in the nutrition count below.

	Calories	Protein	Carbs	Fat	Fiber	Points	Cost
Vegetable Omelet	290	22	34	7	4	7	About
3 sl. bacon	140	9	1	11	0	4	$8.99
Scrambled Egg Whites	50	11	1	0	0	1	
Fruit Dish	45	1	12	0	1	0	

Lasagna and Salad

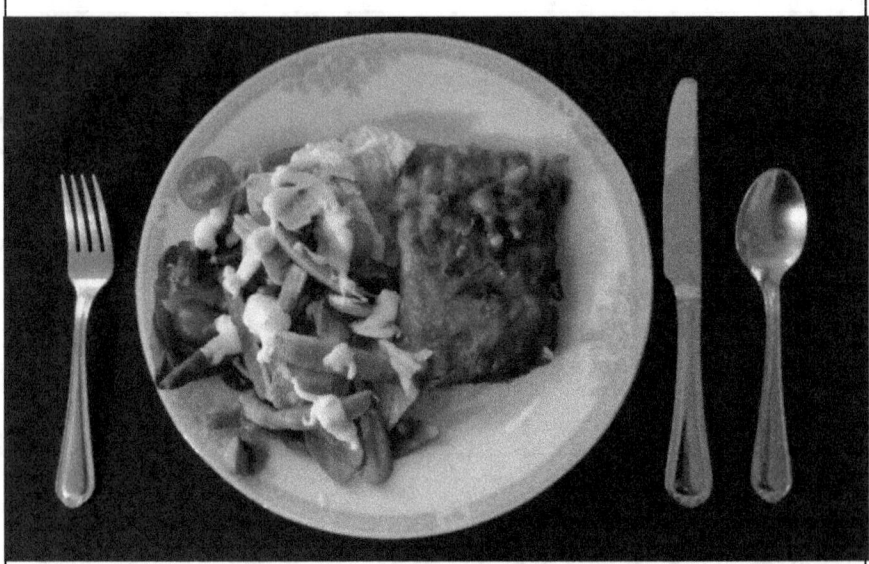

Bremer' Lasagna with Meat Sauce is not a gourmet lasagna, but I find it to be very satisfying when eaten with a tossed salad. Instructions say that you can microwave the lasagna, or cook it in the oven. I prefer the oven. Put it in a 375° oven for one-hour when you get home from work, toss a salad, and your meal is ready.

As you've read before, I'm not a big salad eater so I stopped at a grocery store and bought a small serving of 0-point vegetables from a salad bar—romaine lettuce, mushrooms, red peppers, red onion, snow peas and a tablespoon of green shelled peas. It cost me $2.64, but saved a lot of a bag of salad that would have ended up being thrown out. If you're sharing with a family or friends, of course go the less expensive route. (NOTE: Salad was still more than I wanted so I ate half and saved half for the next day.)

	Calories	Protein	Carbs	Fat	Fiber	Points	Cost
1/4 Bremer lasagna w/meat sauce	220	9	26	9	1	6	0.65
0-point fresh vegetables	30					0	1.32
2 T. blue cheese dressing	130	1	2	13	0	4	0.05

Sharon Kay, M.A., L.U.T.

DINING OUT: *Ruby Tuesday Petite Sirloin, Grilled Zucchini and Spaghetti squash*

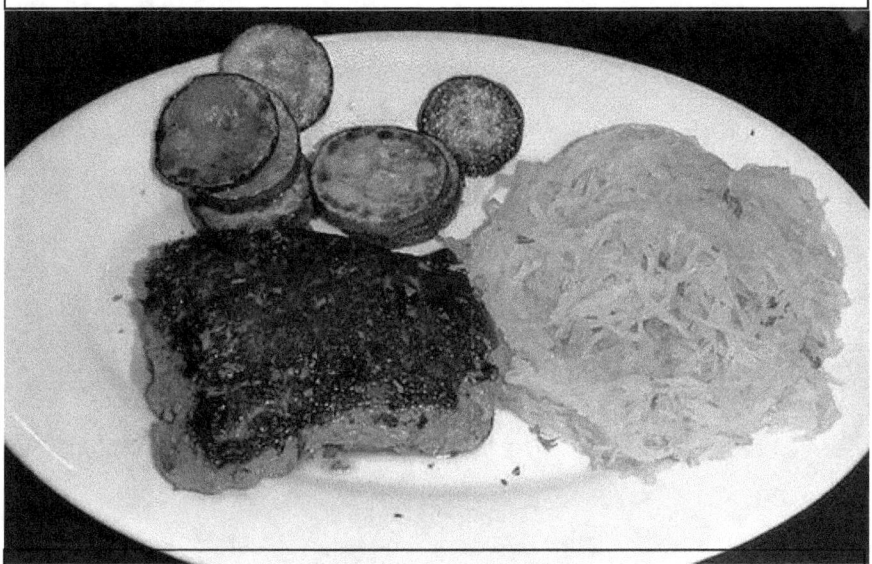

Ruby Tuesday's is another weight-loss friendly restaurant which is a bit more upscale. I usually have this petite sirloin, cooked medium rare, grilled zucchini and well seasoned spaghetti squash.

Their website has "Fit & Trim" items marked in green and, before you leave home, you can search for Ruby Tuesday nutrition and download a PDF file giving nutritional data for everything they serve.

	Calories	Protein	Carbs	Fat	Fiber	Points	Cost
Petite sirloin (7 oz.)	365	35	11	19	3	9	$11.99
Roasted spaghetti squash	41	1	4	2	1	1	
Grilled Zucchini	54	1	6	3	2	1	

Sharon Kay, M.A., L.U.T.

I gave a plate of Vindaloo Chicken, Bhindi Masala and rice to a supervisor and friend yesterday. Her reaction:

I could write it across the sky!
Thanks for the fabulous meal. What a blessing!

Hugs,

Joy

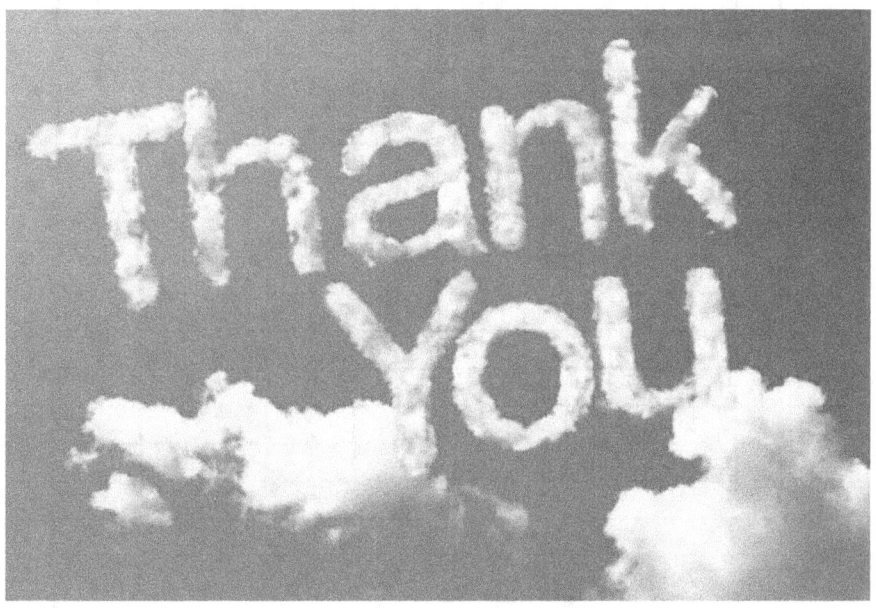

While these meals may seem simple, because they are, they are meals that I would serve to friends or guests with pride.

ADDENDUM 3: Tracking Graph for Weight Loss

WT#	WEEKS IN 20__																	
	1	2	3	4	5	6	7	8	9	10	11	12	13	14	15	16	17	18
	MONTHS																	

Sharon Kay, M.A., L.U.T.

ADDENDUM 4: Tracking Chart for Calories and Points

ITEM	CALORIES	BALANCE	POINTS	BALANCE
DATE: _____		1,200		32
Breakfast				
Snack				
Snack				
Lunch				
Dinner - 6:00 p.m.				

Your calorie and/or points allotment for the day may be different than mine, but the principle is the same. Write in what you plan to eat, figure the calories and/or points, then subtract. My chart, created in WordPerfect, subtracts each line from the balance automatically. You can easily set up the same thing using Microsoft Word, Excel or any program with a table calculations feature.

ADDENDUM 5: Ceremonies and Exercises

Recently I had an occasion to attend a family get together. It wasn't my family, but it might as well have been deja vu—going back to reunions I attended during my first marriage.

A large percentage of the people in my family, and this family, would have been diagnosed by the medical profession as morbidly obese. People for whom standing up from a chair after sitting for awhile is not easy to do.

I have no right to judge. At one time this was me. I left the gathering wondering how on earth I would ever be able to convince any of these people, one of my primary target audiences for this book, that they can change and why they should. If not for themselves, then for their children who are well on their way to following in their parents' footsteps.

One instance of the power of food that I observed was force feeding an elderly woman. Force-feeding is a bit of an exaggeration, but you tell me what you would call the following scenario.

The woman, one of the handful of people I would consider to be a normal size, was in her 80s and obviously a matriarch in the clan. After she ate her dinner she was offered desserts which she declined. A few minutes later a woman, whom I'm told was her daughter, came to her with a plate that had two servings of different desserts on it and stated that different relatives had made the desserts just for her.

Of course, she ate them. I would probably have done the same thing.

Within a few minutes the woman put her head on the table and, thankfully, went to sleep instead of into a coma. The daughter came back to check on her and laughed about her mother probably being tired from all the extra activity that day—or, she said, maybe it was too much sugar.

You won't often hear me swear, but hell! The woman wouldn't have eaten too much sugar if it hadn't been forced on her. It took all I could do to refrain from telling the daughter off.

And yet, in hindsight, I used to be that woman. Remember my story of teasing my daughter about being a rabbit because she enjoyed eating salads when she was young.

I went away from that gathering feeling very depressed about how effective this book would be. Then I realized that: 1) it is not my job to get the book into the hands of people who need it; and 2) my job is to

Sharon Kay, M.A., L.U.T.

write from my heart ... from a place of love and knowledge about the challenges they face.

I was one of the lucky ones who escaped that lifestyle. It wasn't easy. I remember, after finding Weight Watchers, preparing healthy dishes to take to family gatherings and all of the teasing that ensued. It wasn't easy, but looking and feeling good today made it all worthwhile.

One of the tools I have used to release my past is the Burning Bowl ceremony. Once you have accumulated enough information about your reasons for holding onto excess weight, this is a good practice to do. It is quite simple, but also quite effective. You will notice that I use the word "releasing" as opposed to "losing" when talking about weight loss. Psychologically, when we say that we have lost something there is the thought that we need to find it. But we don't. We want to release excess weight to the universe and leave it there.

BURNING BOWL CEREMONY

You probably already have everything you need:

A bowl that will not be affected by fire
A candle
Decorative items such as rocks to put around the candle
Slips of paper (flash paper, which is inexpensive and easily available, is great)

Write any negative emotions about your body or your weight on the pieces of paper. You can do this over a period of time, or in one session, and it is perfectly okay to do more than one bowl burning as new information comes to you.

Some things that I have written in the past include:

I hate the way my butt looks
I am so fat
I have no discipline
I love chocolates
Etc.

These are all things that are absolutely not true today, including loving chocolates! Chocolates are supposed to be every woman's downfall. I prefer white candies like divinity. Saying "I love sweets" would be more accurate.

Once you are satisfied that you've covered everything, set aside time when you can be by yourself, quiet and uninterrupted, turn your cell phone and other electronic devices off, put on soft music if you like and go into a meditative state. By meditative I don't mean a yoga position. I simply mean quieting your mind.

When you are ready, slowly, purposefully, touch the papers, one at a time, to the candle flame. As you touch each paper to the flame say, "You no longer serve any purpose in my life. I release _____ and accept my highest good."

The words "I release _____" constitute a denial. The words "accept my highest good" constitute an affirmation. it is important when denying something to always replace it with something positive. And that is what you have just done.

In the days ahead, watch for your highest good to manifest. It may come in obvious ways such suddenly finding that you have no desire for pastries. On the other hand, my highest good often manifests in riddles. Perhaps it is because as a child I loved mysteries. Often I have to figure out what a message is telling me, but for me this can be fun! Our higher powers speak to each of us in different ways and it is important to learn how to understand those messages.

Automatic Writing

Automatic writing, for those of you who don't feel that communing with your angels or spirit guides is too "woo woo," can be helpful in finding out reasons that you insist on holding on to excess weight.

There are a number of ways to contact these higher beings, but simply sitting still with pen in hand is a fairly quick and easy way.

According to the website www.angels.about.com, "Some people practice automatic writing with angels, which involves channeling an angel and inviting that angel to use the human body to write messages. After asking a question through prayer or meditation, people begin to write whatever thoughts enter their minds without consciously thinking about what they will write.

"Later, when they read those written messages, they say that they may receive angelic insights into whatever topics about which they'd been seeking guidance."

We can obtain information by this method if we choose to do so, and I have, but most of what I share with you has come simply through trial-and-error experience. As with any good mother I hope that you can learn some lessons through my experiences rather than having to make all the mistakes I made.

Sharon Kay, M.A., L.U.T.

_____

_____

_____

_____

_____

_____

_____

_____

_____

_____

_____

_____

_____

_____

_____

_____

_____

_____

_____

_____

_____

_____

_____

_____

_____

_____

_____

_____

_____

_____

Shape Shifter
Crossword Puzzle

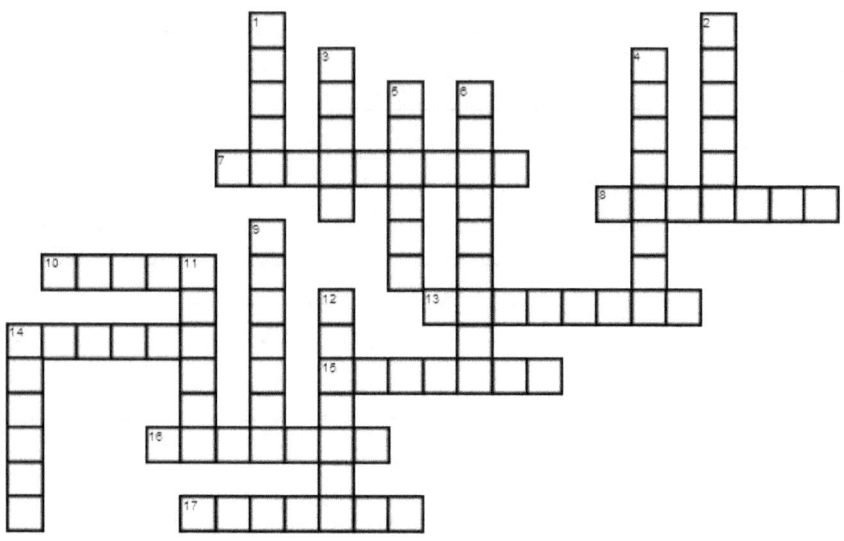

Word games were one of the ways my schoolteacher mother taught me how to read and to expand my vocabulary. I still find them to be a fun exercise and hope that you enjoy this puzzle as much as I enjoyed creating it.

Answers are upside down on the bottom of page 215, but please test your memory on what you have read by trying to answer the questions before looking at the answers.

Crossword created using www.puzzle-maker.com/CW/ program.

Sharon Kay, M.A., L.U.T.

1) Protein and pasta TV dinners can be a quick, easy and nutritious meal by adding a _____ vegetable.

2) I Can't Believe It's Not Butter is a better choice than _____ or margarine.

3) You can eat all the _____ you want.

4) According to the Holmes and Rahe Stress Scale, even _____ events can cause illness (i.e. obesity).

5) All fruit has 0-_____ per serving.

6) Low-calorie bread, fruit and peanut butter make a nutritious _____.

ACROSS:

7) Sugar-free sodas, coffee and tea can be consumed in _____ quantities.

8) Potatoes are a _____ vegetable and a serving is 2-points.

9) _____ oil is one of the most healthy sources of fat.

10) Fresh fruit should be eaten instead of drinking _____ because it is easy to drink too many calories.

11) Exercise will become _____ after you have lost 20-30 pounds.

12) Almond milk contains more _____ than cow's milk.

13) You can track what you eat with _____ or points.

14) An equal amount of _____ cheese is more satisfying than chunk cheese because it appears to be a larger quantity.

15) Grains, even whole grains, should be eaten in _____ quantities.

16) Nuts are a good source of _____, but are high in fat.

17) Most of us do not get enough _____ D.

Let Your Fingers

Do the Walking

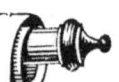

Walking a labyrinth is considered by many to be a spiritual practice. It occurred to me that some of you may not be able at the present time to actually go outdoors and physically walk a labyrinth, or there may not be ne near you.

Use a pencil to follow the labyrinth maze at the right from beginning to end. Do so slowly, meditatively. Repeat an affirmation that you have chosen silently or aloud. Or you may want to listen to the "Shape Shifting Motivational CD" while drawing.

Either way, relax and enjoy the exercise.

Sharon Kay, M.A., L.U.T.

Labyrinth

Meditation

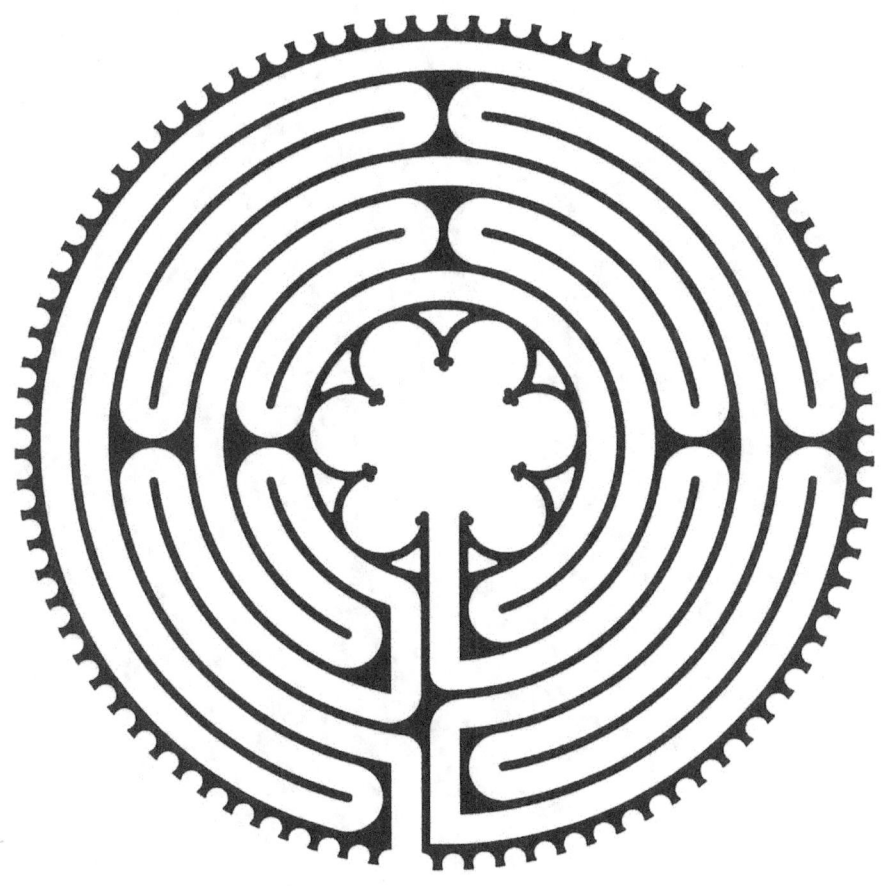

Sharon Kay, M.A., L.U.T.

HOLMES AND RAHE STRESS SCALE

Holmes and Rahe found that a score of 150 gives you a 50/50 chance of developing an illness. A score of 300+ gives you a 90% chance of developing an illness, having an accident or "blowing up." Notice that "positive times" like Christmas, marriage and vacations are stressful.

Multiply event by the number of times you have experienced it in the last year.

	LIFE EVENT (STRESSOR)	VALUE	#/YR	TOTAL
1)	Death of spouse	100 X	___ =	___
2)	Divorce	73 X	___ =	___
3)	Marital separation	65 X	___ =	___
4)	Jail term	63 X	___ =	___
5)	Death of close family member	63 X	___ =	___
6)	Major personal injury or illness	53 X	___ =	___
7)	Marriage	50 X	___ =	___
8)	Fired from work	47 X	___ =	___
9)	Marital reconciliation	45 X	___ =	___
10)	Retirement	45 X	___ =	___
11)	Major change in health of family member	44 X	___ =	___
12)	Pregnancy	40 X	___ =	___
13)	Sex difficulties	39 X	___ =	___
14)	Gain of new family member	39 X	___ =	___
15)	Major business readjustment	39 X	___ =	___
16)	Major change in financial state	38 X	___ =	___
17)	Death of close friend	37 X	___ =	___
18)	Change to different line of work	36 X	___ =	___
19)	Major change in number of arguments with spouse	35 X	___ =	___
20)	Mortgage over $100,000	31 X	___ =	___
21)	Foreclosure of mortgage or loan	30 X	___ =	___
22)	Major change in responsibilities at work	29 X	___ =	___
23)	Son or daughter leaving home	29 X	___ =	___
24)	Trouble with in-laws	29 X	___ =	___
25)	Outstanding personal achievement	28 X	___ =	___
26)	Spouse begins or stops work	26 X	___ =	___
27)	Begin or end school	26 X	___ =	___
28)	Major change in living conditions	25 X	___ =	___
29)	Revision of personal habits	24 X	___ =	___
30)	Trouble with boss	23 X	___ =	___
31)	Major change in work hours or conditions	20 X	___ =	___
32)	Change in residence or schools	20 X	___ =	___
33)	Major change in recreation	19 X	___ =	___
34)	Major change in church activities	19 X	___ =	___
35)	Major change in social activities	18 X	___ =	___
36)	Mortgage or loan less than $10,000	17 X	___ =	___
37)	Major change in sleeping habits	16 X	___ =	___
38)	Major change in number of family get-togethers	15 X	___ =	___
39)	Major change in eating habits	15 X	___ =	___
40)	Vacations, Christmas	13 X	___ =	___
41)	Minor violations of the law	11 X	___ =	___

Score of 300+ = At risk of illness.

Score of 150-299 = Risk of illness is moderate.

Score of <150 = Only a slight risk of illness.

Resources

BOOKS

Bock, Lazlo. *Work Rules!: Insights from Inside Google That Will Transform How You Live and Lead* (New York City: Twelve Publishing Company, 2015)

Buenostar, Laina. *Happy Money* (Self-published eBook, 2012)

Canfield, Jack. *The Success Principles!* (New York City: Harper Collins Publishers LLC, 2004)

Davis, William. *Wheat Belly* (New York City: Rodale, Inc., 2011)

Dispenza, Joe. *You Are the Placebo: Making Your Mind Matter* (New York: Hay House, Inc., 2015)

Fillmore, Charles. *Talks On Truth* (Unity Village, Missouri: Unity Books, 1998)

Fillmore, Charles. *The Twelve Powers of Man (Unity Village, Missouri: Unity Classic Library, 2006.)*

Gawain, Shakti. *Creative Visualization: Use the Power of Your Imagination to Create What You Want in Life* (Mill Valley, California: Whatever Publishing, 1978)

Grout, Pam. *E^3 (New York City: Hay House, Inc., 2014)*

Hay, Louise. *You Can Heal Your Life* (New York City: Hay House, Inc., 2004)

Martella-Whitsett, Linda. *How to Pray Without Talking to God: Moment by Moment, Choice by Choice* (Charlottesville, Virginia: Hampton Roads Publishing Company, Inc., 2011)

Overeaters Anonymous. *Abstinence: Members of Overeaters Anonymous Share Their Experience, Strength and Hope* (Rio Rancho, New Mexico: Overeaters Anonymous Publishing, 1994)

Redfield, James. *The Celestine Prophecy* (New York City: Warner Books, 1993)

Schucman, Helen. *A Course in Miracles* (Mill Valley, California: Foundation for Inner Peace, 2008)

Tipping, Collin. *Radical Forgiveness* (Marieta, Georgia: Global 13 Publications, Inc., 2002)

Tolle, Edkhart. *The Power of Now: A Guide to Spiritual Enlightenment* (Novato, California: New World Library, 1997)

Twyman, James. *The Barn Dance* (New York City: Hay House, Inc., 2010)

Witherspoon, Thomas E. *Myrtle Fillmore: Mother of Unity* (Unity Village, Missouri: Unity Books, 1984)

WEBSITES

www.Abundance-and-Happiness.com
www.CalorieCount.com
www.CompleteWellBeing.com
www.EatingWell.com
www.ForksOverKnives.com
www.Gaia.com
www.HuffingtonPost.com
www.Masaru-Emoto.net
www.MayoClinic.com
www.NaturalRemedies.org/chafing
www.OA.org
www.OrganicFacts.net
Www.Puzzle-Maker.com/CW/
www.TUT.com
www.Unity.org/TwelvePowers
www.WebMD.com
www.WeightWatchers.com
www.Wikipedia.com
www.WineFolly.com

Answers to Shape Shifter Crossword Puzzle"

calcium / 13-calories / 14-grated / 15-limited / 16-protein / 17-vitamin
ACROSS: 7-unlimited / 8-starchy / 9-coconut / 10-juice / 11-easier / 12-

DOWN: 1-green / 2-butter / 3-fruit / 4-positive / 5-points / 6-breakfast

About the Author

Sharon has a passion for people and for living and teaching Unity principles. In living those principles she is Worship Leader at Unity of Independence, Missouri, a Licensed Unity Teacher and actively supports fundraising events for the church.

She holds a Master's degree in Organizational/Developmental psychology and journalism from the University of Houston at Clear Lake, Texas, and trained as a Weight Watchers lecturer in the 70s. She is former Executive Director of a crisis center for abused women and children; wrote for "The Houston Chronicle" newspaper and is author of *Queen for an Hour: A Past-Life Regression* and *Create-A-Miracle PRN (as needed)*. Her website at www.sharonkays.website hosts her blog through which you can ask questions, has up-to-date contact information, and includes information on upcoming speaking engagements, "Loving to Lose" retreats at beautiful Unity Village, Missouri and medical vacations in India.

Contact Sharon

To get the latest *Shape Shifting* updates and resources, visit:

www.sharonkays.website

Sharon speaks frequently on the topic of weight loss. She can deliver a keynote, half-day or full-day version of this content, depending on your needs. If you are interested in finding out more, please visit her Speaking and retreat pages at:

www.sharonkays.website/workshops/

www.sharonkays.website/retreats/

www.sharonkays.website/medical-vacations/

You can also connect with Sharon here:

Blog: www.sharonkays.website

Twitter: www.twitter.com/sharonkay

Facebook: www.facebook.com/sharonkay

WORKSHOPS

What questions do I have? Notes?

_____

_____

_____

_____

_____

_____

_____

_____

_____

_____

_____

_____

_____

_____

_____

_____

_____

_____

_____

_____

_____

_____

_____

_____

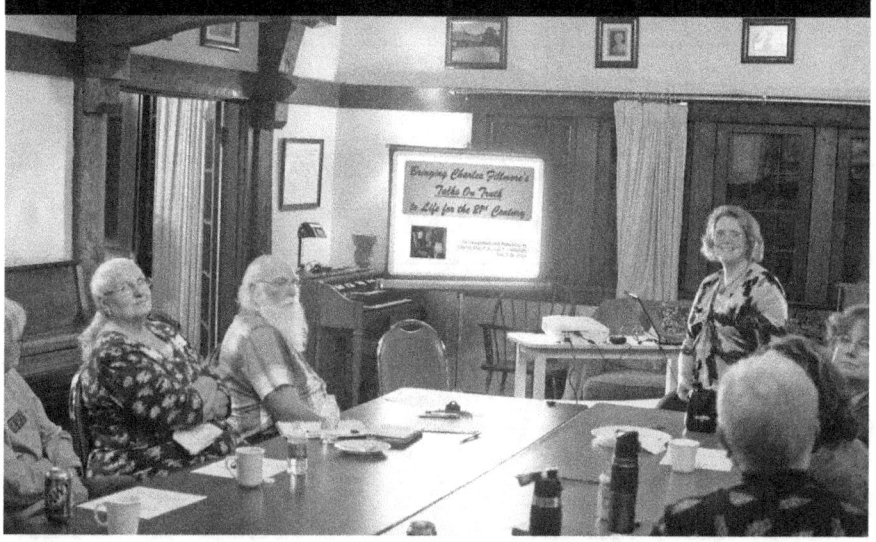

Workshops

Self-Esteem Building

Cooking for Weight Loss

Budgeting: Time/Money/Calories

Creative Visualization

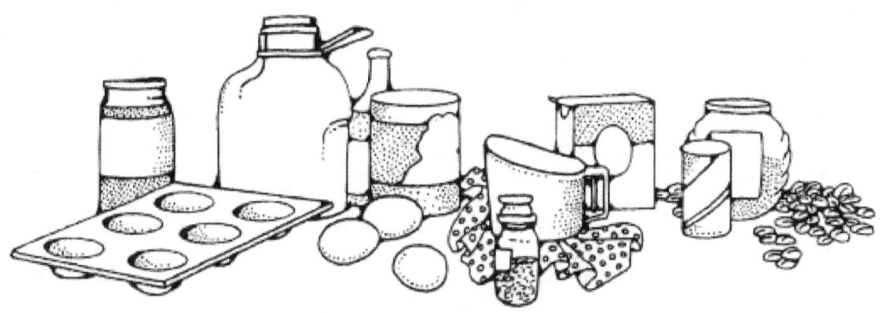

www.sharonkays.website/workshops/

LOVING TO LOSE RETREATS

What questions do I have? Notes?

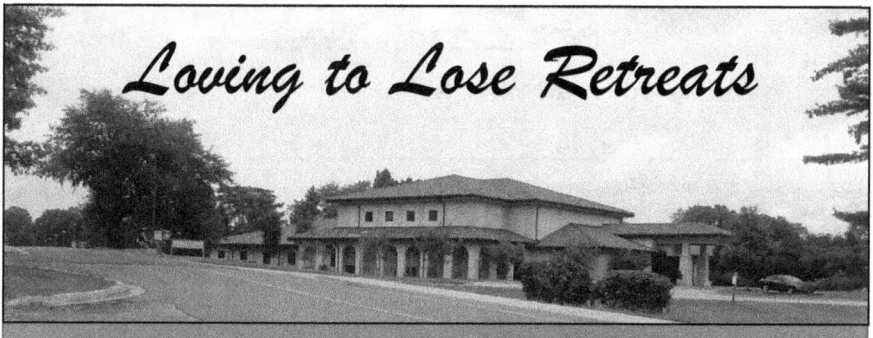

Loving to Lose Retreats

At Beautiful

Unity Village, MO

INCLUDED IN FEE:

Nutrition/Cooking Classes
Gourmet Weight Loss Friendly Meals
Fruit Basket in Every Room
Laughter & Restorative Yoga
Reiki Energy Healing/Drumming Circle

Beautiful Rose Quartz Pendulum w/Class
Fitness Center/Walking Trails/Labyrinth
Private Session w/Sharon

1 Year LTL Club Membership

Social Activities

OPTIONAL EXTRA FEE ITEMS:

Massages
Past Life Regressions
9 Hole Golf Course

www.sharonkays.website/retreats/

MEDICAL VACATIONS IN INDIA

What questions do I have? Notes?

_____

_____

_____

_____

_____

_____

_____

_____

_____

_____

_____

_____

_____

_____

_____

_____

_____

_____

_____

_____

_____

_____

_____

_____

_____

Medical Vacations in India

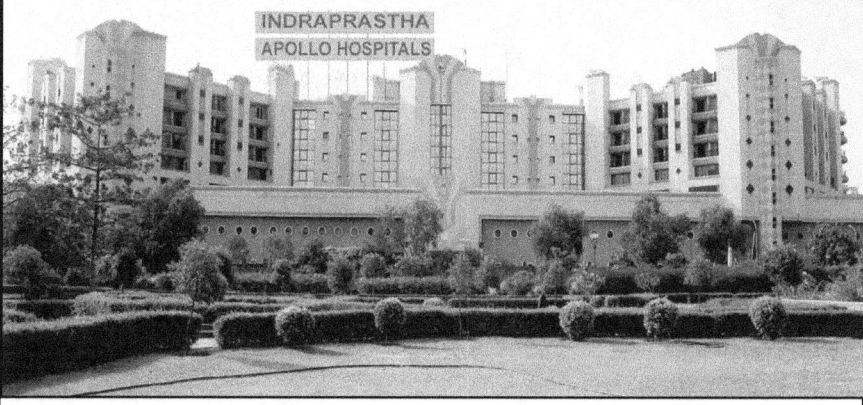

INDRAPRASTHA
APOLLO HOSPITALS

As you have read in this book, Sharon had extensive dental work done in India. Work that would have cost $15,000 in the U.S. cost $1,500 in India. Total expenses, including all items listed below, were less than half what the dental work would have been in Texas.

Two years later Sharon and her husband had executive health assessments done in India—every exam, test or x-ray appropriate for their age and gender—two days of assessments which included consultations with three specialists.

Sharon does not hesitate to have medical procedures done in India and will assist you with all aspects of your healing process.

INCLUDED IN FEE:

Airfare/Ashram or Luxury Hotel
Executive Health Assessment/Massage
English Speaking Guides/Nurses
Meals/Indian Cooking Classes
Reception Party in Indian Home
Historic Excursions, including Taj Mahal
Shopping trips in Marketplace

EXTRA FEE ITEMS:

Medical Procedure(s)
Doctor(s)

www.sharonkays.website/medical-vacations/

Promotional Products for Sale

When I first began showing *Shape Shifter* to friends and colleagues the first thing that caught their eye was the heart and bubbles logo. For Christmas that year I created handmade decoupage ornaments in lavender with the logo. A colleague's husband saw the ornament and asked where they had gotten it. She showed him the book, which she was editing at that time, and he said "That's cool!"

She suggested that it would make a great refrigerator magnet. So I bought magnets to put on the backs of some of these disks which I have come to call "talismans."

Before launching the book I was able to offer:

"I AM Loved" talismans

Ornaments

Keychains

Magnets

Necklaces with silver or rayon cord chains

And now we have the CD on the opposite page. Information on purchase these items can be found on my website at:

www.SharonKays.website/products/

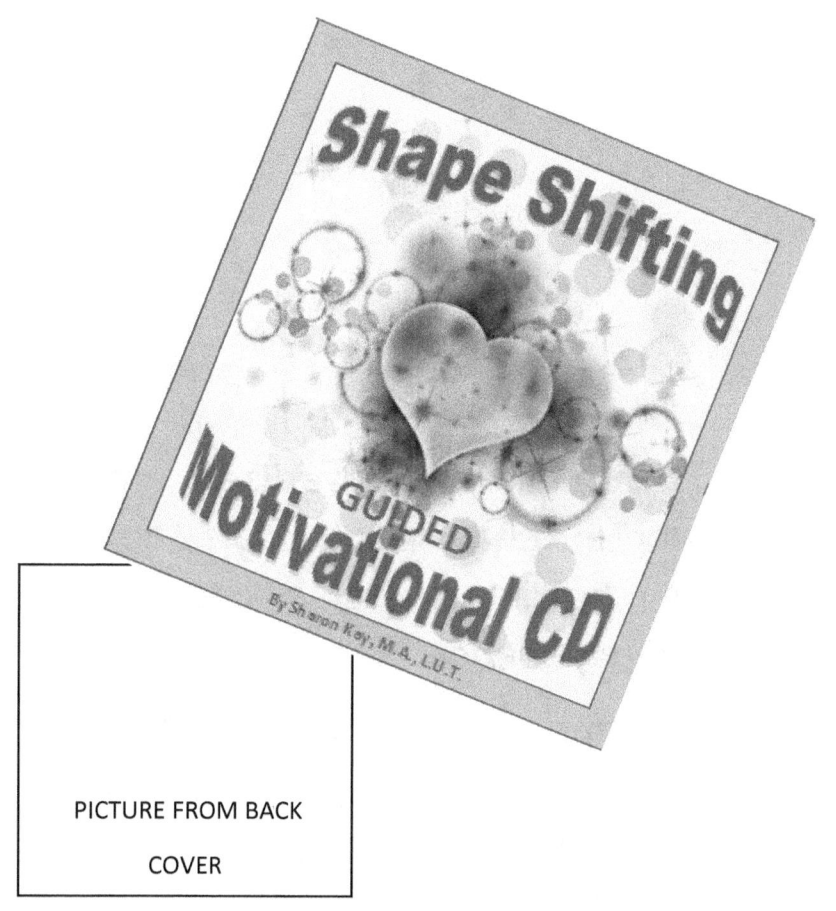

PICTURE FROM BACK

COVER

Find yourself talking with Ascended Masters Jesus the Christ, Mary the mother of Jesus, Sophia the goddess of wisdom and Archangel Raphael ... and your higher self. Walk with them and allow some of the burdens you are carrying to be lifted. They want to help. They are just waiting for you to ask.

Included on the CD is the song "Shaman Woman" written and sung by Gary Johnson, 2007 Iowa Rock & Roll Music Hall of Fame recipient. Based on the true story of Jill Kuykendall, Gary's vision of this remarkable woman who specializes in "Soul Retrieval" assists you in integrating parts of your spirit of which you may not be consciously aware.

CD can be ordered through www.SharonKays.website/CD/ for $5.00 + shipping.

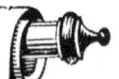

The following advertisers are people I personally endorse for their healing energies, integrity and experience.

Some of them will be working with you when you come to Unity Village for workshops and retreats.

Joy Cherry is a Certified Life Coach through Martha Beck Incorporated and the Q Effect, A Quantum Leap in Living and Leading.

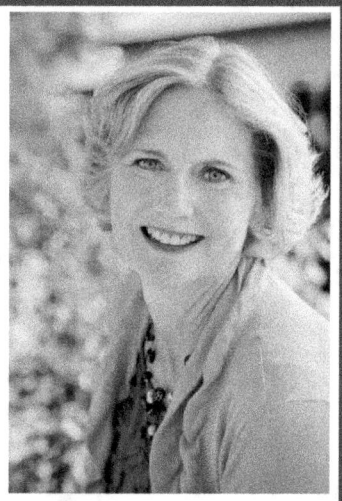

I will help you find your joy riding the river of life and all of its many currents. Using your sense of play and passion I will help you listen to the language of your heart and find your inner inspiration for living your right life.

Prior to life-coaching, Joy was a highly successful financial services operations, management and training professional with a M.A. in Business Management and over 12 years of managerial experience.

www.JoyCherryLifeCoaching.com

joylchr@yahoo.com

816-674-6588

Free 30 minute phone session available by appointment.

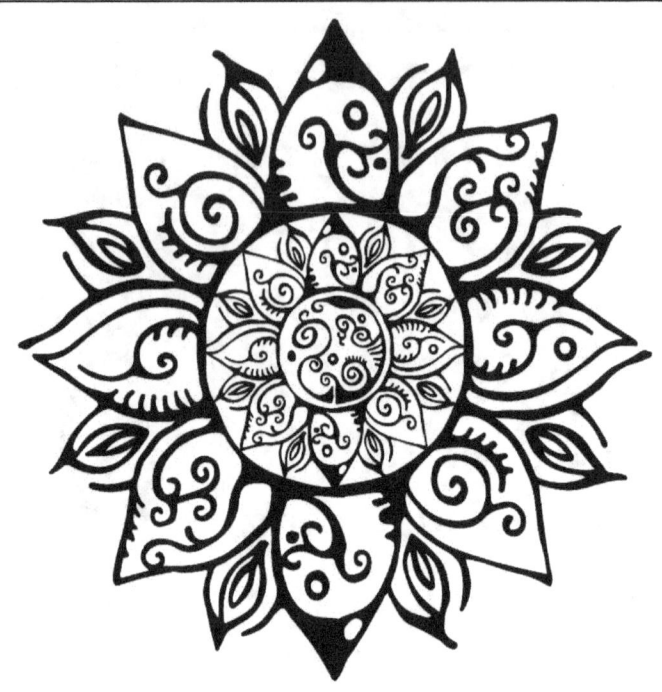

It's Time to Flourish!

Are you ready to live your life more abundantly

with a sense of purpose and passion?

My mission is to "Encourage the flowering of humanity."

Connect with me about my workshops,

classes and one-on-one coaching sessions.

www.RevDianaKennedy.com

816-457-2431

RevDianaKennedy@gmail.com

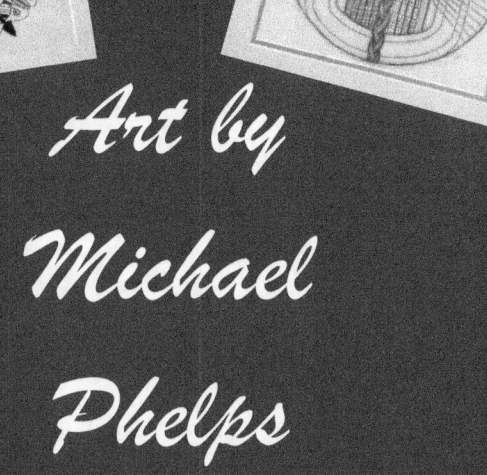

Art by Michael Phelps

My drawings are meditation pieces because you can sit and look at them and see something different every time.

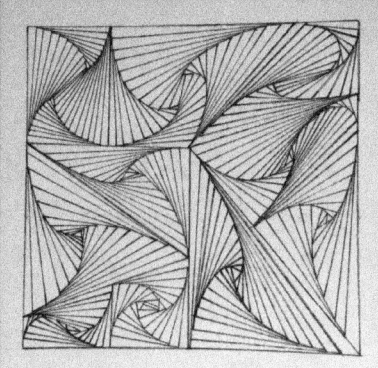